THANK YOU, CANCER

THANK YOU, CANCER

30 DAYS TO REALIZE
NOTHING IS IMPOSSIBLE

LOGAN SNEED

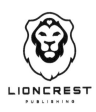

LIONCREST
PUBLISHING

THANK YOU, CANCER

30 Days to Realize Nothing Is Impossible

ISBN   978-1-5445-0502-2 *Hardcover*

          978-1-5445-0501-5 *Paperback*

          978-1-5445-0503-9 *Ebook*

          978-1-5445-0527-5 *Audiobook*

This book is dedicated to my family for experiencing so much so fast! Through the ups and downs, you have been there for me every step of the way. This is also dedicated to every person who has supported me personally through my journey. I want to thank every single one of you for all you have done! The littlest things from liking a photo to leaving a positive comment, and being there every step of the way. I would not be here if it weren't for every single one of you. You have helped me push through every single day in conquering the odds and pushing thousands and millions to do the same.

CONTENTS

"It always seems impossible until it is done..."

—NELSON MANDELA

INTRODUCTION

I'm not exactly known for listening to doctors. Don't get me wrong, doctors have saved my life and given me incredible care through one of the hardest times anyone could go through. But some of them have also told me things like "you have one to ten years to live" and "you won't be able to work out during chemo" and "go have a burger and a beer and enjoy yourself." I couldn't just take their word for it.

However, when one of my doctors saw what I was going through and said, "Logan, you should write a book," I listened. At the time, I wasn't sure how it would all come together. Mostly, I just wanted to have a place to vent while my world was falling apart.

When I was nineteen, in one moment my whole world

changed. I went from high school athlete and college freshman to stage IV glioblastoma patient overnight. I was told to give up on life, on my entrepreneurial dreams...I even lost my girlfriend. The thing is, my life changed for the better just as quickly. It's strange, but the people who doubted me in my life inspired me. My setbacks motivated me to keep going, regardless of what happened.

Nelson Mandela famously said, "It always seems impossible until it's done," and it's true. There is literally no way I could have imagined the obstacles that were ahead of me. There were times when I didn't know how I would get past them. Now that it's done, I'm just grateful.

Writing this book was a challenge. It made me uncomfortable in so many ways. I had to see my story laid out from top to bottom. I had to wrestle with comparison and wonder whether I had anything worth sharing. When I got to the end, I wrote a letter right to cancer. I thought about everything we'd been through together and what I'd learned along the way. I imagined myself stopping the fight, not running anymore, and just turning around to shake cancer's hand and say *thank you* for the way it changed my life.

If you've picked up this book and you're struggling with something—whether you've come here through my fitness channels and you're working on your body, or you're facing cancer or any other obstacle—you have everything you need to overcome it, right there inside of you. I've learned that none of the people who told me "you can't" were ever my obstacle. Really, we make our own limitations.

Think about it. When we're ready to lose weight, if we don't see results after a week, we start to fall off. We tell ourselves that we're failing or that this isn't going to go well. We compare ourselves to other people, hang on to our past, and feed on the negative energy like fuel.

So for the next thirty days, I'd love to share my story with you as you face your own obstacles. Take your time. Use what I've learned along the way as fuel that can keep you going, no matter what you're up against. In fact, as you're reading my story and thinking about your own life, see if you can find a way to actually *thank* that obstacle or struggle.

Think of it this way: Could you write a letter to your weight, your debt, or your business? Could you thank it for making you grow? Can you find room to become happier, to enjoy the present, and to face the fear and doubt that has held you back?

Let's do that together. Let's find the energy, inspiration,

and power to stop saying *f***you* and start saying *thank you* to the stuff in our way.

Thank you for letting me share my story with you. Thank you for taking me along on your journey as you face your own impossible situation. Thank you for giving me some of your precious, beautiful time, and for investing it all into the better you that you're creating every day.

Remember, it only seems impossible until it's done.

INNER FORTITUDE

"Once your mindset changes, everything on the outside will change along with it."

—STEVE MARABOLI, *LIFE, THE TRUTH, AND BEING FREE*

* * *

Pre-Diagnosis

I'm nineteen and wrapping up my freshman year in college. Life is as good as it can possibly be. I have a vision. I want to carve my own path. The very first day of school, I tell my girlfriend of four years that my goal is to drop out one day.

My parents are completely on board, as always. I'd played

basketball all through high school and could have accepted scholarships to play in college, but I wanted to be an entrepreneur. My dad and I started a private-label bodybuilding supplement company, and now it's tracking to become my full-time gig.

As long as I wait until my company is off the ground before quitting, they're completely fine with my plan. Honestly, they've never not been supportive. I think—I know—I'm invincible.

* * *

THOUGHT

noun. an intention, hope, or idea of doing or receiving something.

synonyms: anticipation, expectation, prospect, contemplation, likelihood, possibility.

Nothing bad was ever on my radar. Maybe that made some things go unnoticed, like the mild headaches I would get pretty regularly. But things were too good and my dreams were too big to slow down for something like a headache.

On March 6, 2016, I didn't have a choice anymore.

That morning, I was so motivated. It was time to get lean, hit my bulking goal, shred up for summer. So I prepped a meal, posted a picture on Instagram, and headed out for the gym. On the way there, I FaceTimed my girlfriend, set my phone on my knee, and smiled when I saw her face. I know, I know. Maybe I shouldn't have been on the phone while I was driving. I was just trying to be a good boyfriend. And really, if I hadn't called her, I'm not sure what would have happened.

Within seconds, something went wrong. I knew exactly what I was trying to say, but the words didn't come out. It felt like I was a robot with bad programming or something. My body was doing something completely different than what I thought it should. She thought I was playing a joke on her as I started to slur, but then the seizure started.

She and her mom watched from the phone at my knee as I drove for about a half mile, completely unconscious. If I'd already been on the highway, my story would have ended very differently. Thankfully, I ran into a little ditch and wound up without any damage to the car at all. My girlfriend called an ambulance, and I remember waking up inside of it for just a quick moment. I could tell where I was but had no idea why. A few hours later, I woke up again, this time lying on my side on something like a stretcher. I could hear voices, see the bar of the bed in front of my face and the doctor's jacket on the other side. My mom was there...and then I was gone again.

No one really knew what was going on. They asked all of the standard questions—has he ever had a seizure, is he doing any drugs, does he have any health issues—and had no obvious answers. When I came around, they did some blood work and a CAT scan. Nothing.

The weird thing was, I felt fine once I woke back up. My parents caught me up on everything that had happened, and it just seemed...weird. I didn't feel sick. I didn't feel weak or in pain. It was just a weird thing that happened.

Obviously, a seizure is more than just a *thing*, but I figured it couldn't be that bad if I still felt as good as I did. Maybe I'd over-trained or something; that was it.

My mom and the doctors knew otherwise. She wanted to figure this out, which I guess is just the way a mom works. They agreed I needed an MRI within a day or so. A year later, my mom told me that she and my girlfriend took it hard. While I was getting scanned, she went to the bathroom and broke down crying while my girlfriend sat on the couch in the waiting room, crying as well. They were way ahead of the game. I wouldn't catch up for a while still.

Mostly, I took it all in stride. The odds of having something really bad were so low, this was more about making everyone feel better. Maybe it was even a waste of time. I didn't need answers for a thing that happened once and was over without any damage. I had the life I wanted. I couldn't wrap my mind around anything changing that.

Even when the neurologist told me they saw something on the MRI, I wrote it off. Even when they said it was big enough that we had to go to a neurosurgeon, I couldn't accept it. I didn't even feel like it was active denial—it was an honest belief that nothing that bad could actually happen.

Thoughts are powerful. So powerful that we can completely delude ourselves with them. I'd learned to live in the present, but that's not the same as accepting the present. My thoughts were so far removed from what was actually happening. There I was, meeting with a doctor who was preparing to do surgery on my brain, still thinking I was invincible.

When something challenging is in front of you, from a big goal to a big surgery, accept it. That thing is like the roots of a beautiful tree. You might not have the power to know what it's going to look like on the other side just yet, but that's okay. You have the power to face each moment as it comes. Life is a journey, and all we have is the day that's in front of us. Don't waste time running from reality.

WORDS

noun, plural. speech as distinct from action...a person's account of the truth, especially when it differs from that of another person...a message; news.

If I thought the MRI was a waste of time, the neurosurgery appointment was a nightmare. We were there for something like two hours. I paced in the hall. I sat there on my phone. I was completely irritated at how long we had to wait just to get in to talk to someone about this thing that I was sure would be over any minute now.

When we finally got into the room, the neurosurgeon shook my hand and got right to business: "Good to meet you. It looks like you've got something going on in there. Before we get started, we need to clear some things up..."

The mass was in a tough spot. Surgery would leave me unable to speak or hear. I wouldn't be able to play basketball again. All within about ten minutes. No hope. No faith. No solutions. No rush, even—he told me we could do the surgery within the next couple of weeks, after he came back from vacation with his family. All delivered with a shrug and an "oh well." Nothing to do but sit back and deteriorate.

For him, I was just another job on another day in the life of a neurosurgeon. The words spilled out of his mouth without any thought for how they impacted me. If I'd taken them to heart and accepted his words as truth, I would have had to accept the negative outcomes that he had resigned to. If my parents had accepted them, we would have had to adopt his hopeless mentality.

I'm so grateful that they didn't.

They were just as shocked at his attitude as I was, and as soon as we walked out of his office they were making plans to get a second opinion. My Uncle Fred made a special request to his friend and former presidential candidate Ross Perot, who helped us gain access to a hospital he has heavily supported—MD Anderson, one of the top cancer facilities in the world. Thanks to their support and the blessing of God, we would soon meet with a new brain surgeon who had at least as much mental strength as my parents.

The staff at MD Anderson brought us in within a couple of days, which felt strange in itself. I still wasn't really on board with what was going on. I definitely didn't feel like a cancer patient. From the moment the neurosurgeon opened the door, none of that mattered. He had a completely different demeanor and was ready to get things going. A journey was beginning, and I didn't have a choice but to follow along.

He quickly said, "Would you be ready for surgery? We need to get this moving within thirty-six hours," and when we relayed the other doctor's concerns about loss of speaking and hearing, he interrupted. "Oh, no. If I'm doing your surgery, that will *not* happen."

As much as the first surgeon drained me, this confidence fueled me.

That's not to say it was easy or that I was totally present. The surgeon made me feel good about the idea of surgery, but preparing for it felt more like *The Twilight Zone* than anything. They set the surgery for the next day, gave me a hospital gown to change into, and then the tests began.

I had an MRI, tests for cognitive function, blood tests. They checked to see how I could memorize pictures and letters, and again it all felt like a waste of time. I was shuffled from room to room all over the hospital. At lunchtime, the cafeteria made me feel even more out of place. So many people looked tired and sad and defeated. I had to be the exception. I couldn't be in the same sad situation they were in. I just had to have surgery, that was it.

As much as I wanted that to be true, my body was taking it harder than I wanted to admit. The MRI was my last test for the day, and when I stood up to walk over to the room, I hit the floor. A nurse caught me so that I didn't hit my head when I passed out. As I came to, I could hear a rush of words all around me: "...hungry...another seizure... in shock...blood draw..."

Shock was probably the most accurate guess. My life sped up to a hundred miles an hour overnight, and I was struggling to catch up.

If thoughts are powerful for us, words might be even stronger. The thing about words is that we can use them on each other, for good or for bad. At this stage especially, words seemed to take over my life. I was completely at the mercy of what everyone else was telling me. While the tests before surgery were overwhelming, I'm so glad I was there and not with the first surgeon.

Looking back, I think that he had some pretty heavy limits on himself. When we set those internal limitations, it closes our minds off. We never see what's truly possible. I can't imagine what it would have been like to go through that process with a surgeon who was defeated from the start. If you're trying to remove obstacles as you prepare to face your challenge, start with yourself. What limitations are you hanging on to?

TRUST

verb. believe in the reliability, truth, ability, or strength of; have confidence; hope.

The night before my surgery, I met with the neurologist's assistant. She explained what was about to happen. The tumor was the size of an egg. The surgery would take seven or eight hours. I would be strapped down so that I couldn't move at all. About halfway through, they would have to wake me up to check on my ability to speak and hear, then they would put me back to sleep until the surgery was over.

I'm not really sure how you're supposed to wrap your mind around something like that. The surgeon's confidence helped. The way they prepared me helped. But there was no way for me to fully comprehend what was about to happen.

All I knew was that my surgeon, Dr. Raymond Sawaya, had it under control. His presence alone brought confidence to everyone in the room. He never doubted himself, and it showed up in his tone and the way he carried himself. I met with the rest of the team one last time before surgery, they put some stickers on my face, and sent me home for the night.

Stepping out of the hospital felt like a freedom I hadn't experienced before. My family and my girlfriend and her family went out to dinner, and except for the stickers on my face, we were just normal people hanging out. There were some thoughts in the back of my mind about how things could go wrong. I could technically still lose my hearing or sight. I could even die, I guess. But I had a great surgeon. I was about to get this thing out of my head...and I was still alive right then. We weren't somber or sad—it was more like a celebration.

At five the next morning, it was a little harder to ignore what was happening. I thought about where my surgeon was and if he was sleeping well. Dark little thoughts popped up, like what if he had a twitch in his hand or had to go to the bathroom? One wrong move could be it for me. Instead of giving in to the doubts, I treated it like a game day. I grabbed some earbuds, picked out some reassuring songs, and we headed out for the hospital. I still get chills thinking about that drive, looking out into the dark morning, taking in the lyrics, "If God is with us, what could stand against us?" Preparing for the worst and hoping for the best.

When we walked into the hospital from the parking garage, we went to a lobby area where each family had their own section to wait in before the patient was taken through the hallway and to their pre-op room. The lights were dimmed. Some people were sleeping. Others were crying. Patients were changing clothes and climbing onto their stretchers. When it was my turn to change and lie down, a small group gathered around me. The chaplain, my girlfriend, and both of our dads stood there and prayed over me, and then it was time to say goodbye.

They wheeled me away from my girlfriend and family while she sobbed behind me, and it felt like being dragged off to my own funeral. The hallway was like something out of a dream or a sci-fi show. Nuclear warning signs were on every door; the walls were thick with glass that looked bulletproof. You'd think they were making bombs, not saving people. Meanwhile, the people pushing my stretcher tried to make conversation, like we were good friends about to have a great time.

I didn't see the surgeon before we got started, but I knew he was coming. The operating room was like something out of a movie, with lights and tools and something like a huge tube in the middle of the room. Up above us there were so many doctors, all looking down from a control room like they were offensive coordinators at a football game. Nurses were lined up around the room in their masks, waiting to get started. They explained the anesthesia to me, and then I was gone.

What seemed like minutes later, I was awake again, fully aware that this was the mid-surgery test they'd prepared me for. I wanted to answer their questions thoroughly and confidently so that they knew there was still hope. So that they didn't give up on me. They asked me my brothers' names and hobbies, what kind of sports I played and what school I went to. I still couldn't see my surgeon, but I knew his hands were in my exposed brain right then. I knew I could hear and see and that we were on the right track. He just had to keep going and get that mass all the way out. They put me back to sleep, and when I woke up again it was over.

One little mistake could have been a disaster, and I had no control over it at all. There was nothing I could do to make it better or easier for the doctors. All I could do was take one moment at a time until I made it through to the other side. My trust in the surgeon was teaching me how to trust God and come to accept the present moment.

If you're being hit with negative influences and doubt and disbelief from other people, it will feed disbelief in yourself. Take a look at your influences. If you're struggling to remove self-limitation, maybe there are some other voices you need to get rid of too. Surround yourself with people who you can trust and who inspire you to love and accept your life no matter what happens.

PAIN

noun. physical suffering or discomfort caused by illness or injury.

synonyms: suffering, affliction, discomfort.

Right after surgery, it seemed like every five minutes someone was asking me, "How do you feel?" *How do I feel? I feel* angry; *that's how I feel!* As much as the team tried to prepare me for the surgery, I thought that was going to be the worst of it. When it was over, I would get up and get back to my summer workout plans. Instead of this awful interruption being over, I woke up to pain.

There wasn't really any pain at the site of the surgery. It was more like random pinches and twinges all over my body. No one ever died from a pinch, but it was the most annoying form of pain you can imagine. To make things worse, I couldn't even see my family right away. As much as I wanted out, my nervous system had to take time to recover from the shock we'd just given it. I was stuck in a room by myself for hours while everyone asked me how I was feeling. I felt annoyed. I felt angry. I felt stuck. I felt like I couldn't control myself. I felt like I wasn't prepared for any of this. I just wanted it to be over.

Within a day or so, I was able to take my first steps out of the room, to everyone's surprise. The nurses helped me get through those first days of recovery, and before I knew it I was back in the cafeteria, crazy bandages, half of my head shaved and all. I remember sipping on a smoothie and looking around, just like I had before the surgery, but this time I felt like I fit in a little bit more. Could I really be part of this? Was I just a dude observing people in a sad situation, or was I in one of them too?

The surgeon told me the whole mass was removed, and when it was time to go home again, I wanted to feel as invincible as I had before. But there were scars and markers telling me otherwise. My hair still had to grow back. I had to keep my head elevated for about a week, so I slept on the couch. I couldn't work out any heavier than a walk on the treadmill for another twelve weeks. My body felt like mine, but my recovering brain felt like a torn map. I couldn't get all the way back to the life I had before.

From the first day home, I felt so supported by people around me. When I couldn't feel invincible anymore, so many people stepped up to remind me just how much I had been through already. I was the guy who just had brain surgery and wanted to get back to the gym. It felt good and motivated me to keep going. To keep pushing toward my dreams.

I had no idea what was still to come. None of us really do. Especially when your roadmap changes suddenly, it's hard to wrap your mind around what's happening. The thing is, it's okay to not know. Accept your reality, for whatever it is, and decide to take it on. Grab on to the people who are cheering you on when you don't feel like you can do it on your own. Together, you can take this new path to your goals. You can start to move forward in spite of the discomfort, loss of control, and setbacks.

DESPAIR

noun. the complete loss or absence of hope.

synonyms: distress, anguish, pain, unhappiness.

Ten days after surgery, still a few days before we were supposed to meet with the surgeon about the biopsy results and official diagnosis, my mom called me into the office. We'd all been watching a basketball game late at night, but at some point my mom and dad disappeared into the other room. They looked pretty serious. I honestly thought I might be in trouble for something, there was that kind of feeling in the room. But then my mom explained what happened. That night, completely out of the blue, she'd gotten an email from the hospital, followed quickly by a call.

They'd sent my diagnosis by mistake. Stage IV glioblastoma—a severe form of cancer that was nearly impossible to treat, but they would do everything they could.

The nurse called as soon as she'd realized what happened and apologized for the mistake. This wasn't how we were supposed to find out. Mistake or not, this wasn't the news I was supposed to get at all.

I slouched back onto the couch and sank deeper into my reality than I had before. This wasn't just going to go away. This wasn't simple. I wasn't invincible.

A few days later, we met with the neuro-oncologist. While I'd hoped she would give me some answers or let us know it wasn't as bad as the nurse had said, she had no good news for me. She really didn't even want to look me in the eye. She explained that I had one of the most deadly cancers out there. She told me that it absolutely would come back—it was just a matter of when. That no matter what we did, I would only have another ten years to live at most, maybe as little as one year.

My parents asked all the questions. They asked what caused it. They asked what chemo and radiation would be like. They asked what else we could do beyond those treatments. The doctor didn't have answers or strategies for us. I remember my dad asking, "Are you telling my son that he should go have a beer and a burger and wait to die?" and the doctor saying *yes*.

I couldn't talk, couldn't move. Anything I'd ever heard about living positively and choosing good thoughts felt hollow. All of the encouraging words from friends and family and followers were stripped away by the level of hopelessness in that room.

The diagnosis left me in a fog. I couldn't sleep. I would sit in the corner of my room in the middle of the night, bawling my eyes out, alone in the dark. I could handle being the guy who had brain surgery, but this was something different. Why were we even trying? What was the point of me being here if there was no hope anyway? One year, ten years, did it really make a difference? Who would want to be part of my life when so little of it was left?

Everything that I'd preached to myself and others about overcoming the odds wasn't enough to meet these odds.

The "smile and be happy" advice that I'd always clung to wasn't enough. I didn't realize there were deeper lessons to be learned. Life wasn't always going to get better. I couldn't just wait it out and ignore the hard times until they went away. I had to face them and deal with the anger and grief that came with them. If I'd stayed in denial, I wouldn't have been able to create the life that I have.

My good friend Brandon Hawk says that we have to accept the bad stuff in our lives in order to move on from it. Things really can always be worse. It doesn't matter. What matters is that we accept whatever is here and now and prepare ourselves to face it head on.

DETERMINATION

noun. firmness of purpose; resoluteness.

e.g. "he advanced with an unflinching determination"

I didn't care about how I got cancer. I wanted to know how to get rid of it. When the numbness wore off, I found anger waiting for me. Who was the neuro-oncologist to tell me how long my life was going to be? She wanted me to take my prognosis and just wait around for death, and I could have believed her. The phrase "one to ten years" followed me around like a cloud, every moment of every day. I had two options: listen to that voice—go have a burger and a beer and wait for death—or learn to adjust to my new life in spite of it.

Thankfully, my parents had been searching for solutions

already. We met with a new doctor who prepared me for chemotherapy and radiation. Because of the way this type of cancer works, we had to treat it as though there might be some pieces of the tumor left in there, even though it looked like the whole thing had come out. This doctor also gave me a bleak outlook. He said I was going to sit back with the drugs in my system and hope for the best, likely with fatigue, nausea, and all kinds of horrible side effects. The handful of chemo pills next to my dinner plate seemed wrong. I had no idea if they were helping or hurting me.

Radiation would be difficult too. The ward felt like a roomful of zombies, and I was one of them. Some couldn't walk. Some had lost a bunch of weight. The room was silent except for the patients who were struggling to breathe. I also noticed how much older everyone else in the waiting room was. One woman across from me asked something I'd asked myself so many times before: "What are *you* doing here?"

When the nurse walked me back through thick barricaded doors full of warning signs about radiation, I followed her. When they strapped me into the bed and secured the mask to protect the rest of my head from the radiation, I tried to breathe and concentrated on the smooth jazz playing behind the noisy machines—tried *not* to think about everyone else protecting themselves from the thing hitting my brain.

Forty-five minutes later, I stepped out of that first treatment with a new sense of confidence. I was doing what I had to, and my parents had my back. They took me to treatments. My mom and my girlfriend would sit in the waiting room and would drive me home. My dad looked into nutritional options. Even though I was alone physically and would experience some isolation down the road, I was never really on my own.

What was I doing there, really? Maybe I didn't think I belonged there. Maybe no one belongs there. But now that it had happened, I had to take it one step at a time. Their strength got me through.

We all have two voices in our heads, and a choice of which one to listen to. There's doubt and hope. Hell and heaven. Failure and success. Defeat and reassurance. Whichever voice we listen to is the direction we'll move toward. If your vision, habits, or lifestyle are stuck, think about the voices you're listening to. Who is controlling you? Who's going to win?

GROWTH

noun. the process of developing or maturing physically, mentally, or spiritually.

synonyms: expansion, progress, advancement, furtherance

My first lesson had finally become clear: God was telling me that I was never going to achieve my goals on my own. Radiation was happening every day, Monday through Friday, for thirty days—and school was still in session. My mom and I stayed in a little apartment near the hospital for that month, and I'd go to classes and see my friends and girlfriend when I could. I tried to work with the professors but no one was really cutting me much slack. It was a lot to work through, and there was no way I could do it all on my own, not to mention the goals I had for my body and my business. If I wasn't going to just sit back and take my prognosis and lean into the side effects, I would have to rely on God and lean on my family.

Over and over again, experts were telling me that I wasn't any different than anyone else. I was going to struggle just as much, if not more, because of the disease and necessary treatment. It started to piss me off. It started to fuel me. I could accept that I had an awful disease, but I didn't have to let it control me. I couldn't let it destroy me.

For twelve weeks after surgery, I had to take it easy. As soon as that time was up, I grabbed the surgical mask I wore everywhere and headed out for the gym. At first I just walked and let my body readjust to exercise slowly. I watched to see how I would feel or react since I was still in the middle of treatments. When nothing bad happened, I moved on to some lifting. Slowly and steadily, I got back to the things I'd been doing before.

Two weeks into chemotherapy, we met with the doctor for him to check in on my progress. He asked, "How are you? I know it's difficult to not work out while you're on chemo. Are you doing okay?"

I was proud to answer, "I feel great, and I can work out!"

He said, "No, I know it's difficult, but you won't be able to."

With his preconceived ideas about what my experience would look like, it was hard for him to understand what I was saying. Not only was I back in the gym, but I was seeing results. My body was getting leaner and healthier, and my endurance was picking up. Before long, I was riding my bike through the city to get to the gym and then completing my workouts.

At the same time, we'd made research a family project, in a way. Everyone wanted to figure out what else we could do. I think in a way, we wanted to keep proving the doctors and their doubts wrong. If I could put on a germ mask and go work out when they told me it was literally impossible, what else could I do? I started drinking only alkaline water. I changed my shampoo. Nothing had to cure cancer on its own, but if I could make a choice that would help me live a month longer or a year longer, maybe all of those choices would snowball into something significant. It didn't hurt to try.

I wasn't dropped into the middle of this life I have today. I didn't feel great every day or have a thriving business right away. It took time to get there, and it started with these small steps along the way.

One of the biggest setbacks you'll face is if you never get started at all. So many of us get trapped mentally, emotionally, and physically—and we're only at the starting line! Rome wasn't built in a day, right? People don't make big businesses in a day. People don't get past these giant hurdles in life in a day. If you're going to overcome something big, you have to take that first step. Start somewhere. Start *anywhere*. Those baby steps will lead you to the new version of yourself that you've been looking for.

FORWARD MOTION

"We keep moving forward, opening up new doors and doing new things, because we're curious...and curiosity keeps leading us down new paths."

—WALT DISNEY COMPANY

* * *

Post-Radiation

Radiation is finally over. I've got a few weeks left of chemo, and I'm still feeling good—good enough to go out to the river with my mentor, Chad, for the afternoon.

Out in the sun on paddleboards, we talk about the future

and what on earth has happened to me over the last couple of months. I tell him I'm doing everything I can to take care of my body and prevent regrowth, but that the doctors are telling me there's nothing I can do. He tells me about keto.

I think this might be something I can do.

* * *

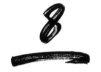

POTENTIAL

noun. having or showing the capacity to become or develop into something in the future.

synonyms: in the making, unrealized, undeveloped

Chad and I met on social media back when I needed a trainer for basketball. His guidance shaped me as an athlete, but I had no idea how much he would influence my life that one weekend on the river. More than anything, he just listened to me. He let me vent about my experience, talk through my thoughts, and relay my fears. There were so many unknowns ahead of me, more than I'd ever thought possible. Everything I thought I knew about my life had been stripped away. I was almost done with chemo, but I still had seizure medications, regular

MRIs, and this looming sense that death could be around any corner.

When I stopped venting, Chad asked me a question that would change my life, finally for the better. He asked, "Have you ever heard of the ketogenic diet?"

Chad told me about a trip that he'd taken to Hawaii where he met a bunch of people following this diet. He explained that it followed high fat, medium protein, low carb intake, and that eating a lot of fat could actually cause your body to lose fat. Because our bodies use sugar as fuel, if we don't eat sugars then our bodies have to find another source of fuel—like body fat.

The reason he thought of me, he went on to explain, is because cancer uses sugar as fuel as well. He wasn't sure what those implications really were, but he thought I might want to look into it.

Finally! After weeks of researching and trying to grab on to some hope, I finally had something to research. I stayed up until one that morning learning about the keto diet and matching it against what I'd learned about brain tumors. I researched how it pertained to my fitness goals, then stumbled upon how it might help with the seizures that my doctor said I'd always have. There weren't many people talking about keto on social media and in the fitness realm yet, but it had been around for a while. Everything seemed to check out, and when I woke up the next morning, I dove right in.

Honestly, it didn't matter how new or odd it felt. My life was on the line, which meant I had no room for flight mode. I had to fight this thing in any way possible, which for now looked like cutting carbs and upping fat intake.

The more I learned about keto, the more convinced I was that I had to do it. The research around epilepsy in kids made it super clear to me. That's actually where keto came from—it was the standard treatment for kids with epilepsy before medication was developed. And it worked.

The doctors had told me I would have seizures once a month and that I had to take temozolomide regularly to prevent them. After months of chemo pills, I was tired of taking medication. If I could take care of the seizures without adding more poison into my body, that's what I was going to do.

The next time I saw my doctor, I told him I was going to stop taking that medication. I explained what I was doing and how sure I was that it was going to work. He wasn't thrilled, but what could he really do? I'd found a path I could take. Something I could actively do that might make a difference. That was the push that I needed to keep going—not just day to day anymore, but finally back on track toward my dreams.

There's a time for baby steps, and there's a time for jumping in with both feet to take massive action. When you have a vision for something and you know it's possible, go for it. It helps to have nothing to lose, for sure, but don't wait for that moment.

Get a vision, go after it with everything you've got, and never let anything slow you down. The baby steps can show you what's possible, but it's consistency and the courage to make big changes that will really get you over your obstacle or to your dream. Look for the bigger picture and execute toward it every day. That's how you make big things happen.

CHANGE

verb. make or become different.

Change is never easy, whether you've chosen it or it comes up suddenly—or in my case, both. With my life suddenly so much different than it had been earlier that year, people started to take notice. Not only was there the cancer and surgery recovery, but my approach to fitness had changed completely too. People took notice. They didn't just see my results, either. They could see my behavior changing too.

I was back on campus when I started keto, which meant I couldn't go out to eat with everyone else. Instead, I'd prep all of my food in my apartment and eat there or bring it with me. It could have been difficult to stand out or feel left out, but honestly, I was too determined to care. When

I thought of the positives—I got to eat so many delicious foods and still feel great about it—and reminded myself why I was doing it, I didn't struggle with the transition at all. I was just excited!

The most difficult, most visible change I had to make was in my business. When I compared my own life and health standards with what I was selling, I just couldn't do it anymore. The shift meant that I couldn't take the supplements I was selling. So while I'd already been able to value my health above cravings or fitting in, now I had to value it above money too. When I thought about it, I'd been in it for the business alone. It wasn't really bettering my health. If I couldn't take the supplements, how could I tell somebody else to take them? I was creating a brand-new life, and it would require a brand-new business.

I'd been worried about selling my business, but once I did, it felt like a weight off my shoulders. I got rid of that feeling of being fake, even though it cost me the success I'd been counting on. If I hadn't been able to let that business go—if I hadn't decided to be authentic and to help people rather than just going after money—I wouldn't be where I am today. Basically, it took a couple of steps backward before I could make giant leaps forward to my dream of being an entrepreneur.

Within minutes of selling my supplement company, the

name FusionLean came to me. In stepping back, I could see my way forward.

The vision to achieve my goals outweighed any fear of failure, even when it looked like I was going in the wrong direction. By hanging on to my vision, it was easier to get past the doubts and second-guessing. I had to stay committed to my health or I would die, and I was committed to staying focused on my dreams until the day I die.

When you catch those fears and uncertainties floating through your mind, redirect them. Intentionally turn your thoughts around. You're not losing something you've had—you're making room for something you want. Something you need. Don't let anyone, not even yourself, tell you otherwise.

OPPORTUNITY

noun. a set of circumstances that makes it possible to do something.

synonyms: time, occasion, moment, opening, window

Without any kind of nausea or side effects during chemo and radiation (except for some mood swings), I had still lost fifty pounds from the time it all started until I was a few months into my new keto lifestyle. It wasn't weight loss from being sick either. I was leaner, fit, and loving my results. I was seeing visible effects of my body using fat as fuel instead of storing it. In spite of the surgery and everything else, I'd achieved the full-body change that I'd wanted back when I was meal planning on the morning of my seizure.

All along the way, I documented what I was doing and how my body was changing. At first people were wishing me well after surgery. Then they were curious about the changes I was seeing. My platforms took off, and before I knew it, I had tens of thousands of people following my updates, for better or worse. With the concept of Fusion-Lean fresh on my mind and a growing following of people who were curious about my new lifestyle, I decided to just launch it and see what happened.

The thing is, I was doing the complete opposite of everyone else. I was eating foods no one ate, avoiding foods everyone said I should eat, and exercising when doctors said I wouldn't be able to. Yet I had all of these results that everyone wanted. It was like living on a different planet. I could have let that loneliness torture me from the beginning. Instead, I invited people to join me on this strange planet. If I could do it while fighting cancer, more and more people believed they could do it too.

I opened up a Wix page and put together a website with some basic information about keto and some PDF files of meal plans based around what I was eating—and that was it. My grandfather was my very first customer. He ordered a simple meal plan and workout plan. But then someone else bought one, and someone else...before long, it snowballed. People came to me for information because of my results, but they stayed and shared it with others because they were seeing results too.

My income quickly hit $1,000 a week, which meant I was close to my original plan to be self-sufficient. I had a whiteboard in my apartment where I tracked daily sales and counted them toward my goals. The more excited I got, the less I could pay attention to my college classes.

A new chapter of my life was beginning, and I couldn't wait to get there. Keto was a complete 180 on my lifestyle and my business. Not only was my body using fat as fuel, but my mindset was fueled by hope and purpose. I'd gotten out of my comfort zone and survived, and that took me to another level of energy, excitement, and motivation.

I wasn't sure what FusionLean would do, but I knew it fit within my vision of becoming a fitness coach. By embracing the strange new life that had been thrown at me, I was able to bring more people onto my journey, and it changed my life.

Johann Wolfgang von Goethe once said, "Courage is the commitment to begin without the guarantee of success." If you're approaching your life with vision and purpose, opportunities will become clear. Take them! What do you have to lose?

CHALLENGE

noun. a task or situation that tests someone's abilities.

I told my girlfriend how close I was to my dream of dropping out and moving to downtown Austin. I dreamed with her about how we could go together. Before long, my focus was fully on my business, even though I still had to stay in college until I could support myself. When one of my professors assigned us a paper on our life goals, I knew exactly what to talk about. Sparked by the excitement I'd found in my new healthy lifestyle and my growing business, I wrote about my vision for the future and turned it in with pride.

I'd been specific about my business and how I saw it growing, but my professor wasn't impressed. She told me how unrealistic it was to talk about being an entrepreneur. She told me I should have been more realistic. She doubted that I could do what I'd written about. Then she gave me a fifty—almost low enough to fail the whole class.

I was livid.

I stormed out of the room, got back to my dorm, and slammed the door behind me. Why could she doubt me like that? Was she doubting herself too? She had her own business on the side, why couldn't I run my own too?

I emptied my backpack out and spread everything around the room. I threw books against the wall, stomped around, and basically lost my cool entirely. Call it chemo mood swings, call it what you will, but my girlfriend walked in right then. I told her what had happened—*she told me to write about what I wanted to do, then freaking failed me on it!*—while she listened and tried to calm me down.

It just felt so personal. It felt…it felt like the doctors telling me the surgery was going to suck, the effects would be horrible, the treatment would be miserable, I wasn't going to win…I was going to die. I should just lie back and accept it. Why try anything at all?

Here I thought I was the CEO of my own life, when challenges from other people could throw me into a spiral like that. The truth was, I wasn't angry because I felt like they were wrong. I was angry because some part of me believed them.

When they told me I would die within ten years, when they told me I'd become a failure...they were saying out loud what I was most worried about. My challenge wasn't to disprove them, but to change my own beliefs. The only way someone else can influence you that much is if you let them. Their doubts—*my own* doubts—were as dangerous for my mindset as the tumor was for my brain.

What was reality telling me? Surgery wasn't what we were afraid it would be. Chemo wasn't as bad as we thought it would be. I actually *did* have a way to be proactive—keto was making a difference. And my business was actually taking off. That's what I needed to latch onto. I needed to treat my mindset like fuel, just like I did with my body and food. I never wanted to be in college in the first place, and I was done being held back by it. I didn't want my professor to be the CEO of my life, just like I didn't want that from the doctors who had such a bleak outlook. I wanted to listen to myself, to be my own CEO. Maybe I drew the short end of the stick and didn't have all the best advantages to get where I wanted to go. But I could use what I had. I could still build the life I wanted.

I told my girlfriend I was ready to drop out and that she could come with me. We could focus on the business together and make a living right then. Or she could stay and I could build the business until we were ready to get married. Real life—the life I'd dreamed of, in spite of all the setbacks—was just around the corner.

My path hasn't been easy. It's been pretty treacherous. Being in denial didn't help me, but neither did hanging on to doubts. If I wanted to accomplish the uncommon—beating cancer, becoming an entrepreneur—I had to think in uncommon ways. I had to get uncomfortable. I had to keep my eyes on the prize and never slip off of the path.

As humans, we become our thoughts. Our actions come from our beliefs. When we see hopelessness, we internalize it. We make it our own. Challenging your own beliefs is never comfortable, but sometimes that's what's necessary. Check to see whether those opinions are fears that you haven't fully faced. Until you deal with them in your own heart and mind, you won't be able to deal with them coming at you from other people.

CONNECTION

noun. a relationship in which a person, thing, or idea is linked or associated with something else.

synonyms: relationship, interconnection, interdependence, attachment, bond

My girlfriend had been amazing throughout the whole cancer journey. She came to treatments and tests, stayed by my side, and stuck with me when I stuck out from the crowd with my masks and diet. We'd been together for four years, and every morning, we'd start our day off with texts about how grateful we were for each other and for our relationship.

One morning, I woke up to a very different kind of text.

The night before, we'd been hanging out watching movies, and that day we had plans to go to a football game with some other people. Out of the blue, she sent me this long text explaining why we needed to break up.

I'd known that we weren't quite on the same page with my business and future plans, but I didn't think we were that far gone. Honestly, I didn't see it coming at all. She had been one of the biggest supporters in my life, definitely the biggest supporter outside of my family. And now she was gone. I couldn't even reach her on the phone. Couldn't see her. I think if we'd seen each other it would have been harder for her and she just wanted to get past it. But I couldn't deal with the fact that we didn't just break up—I'd lost her completely.

I tried to deal with what was happening, but I didn't have anyone to turn to. My roommate was out of town. My parents were at home in Austin. Outside of them, I had no other friends or support. For anything else, I would have turned to my girlfriend. But she wasn't my girlfriend anymore, and I was sure she was out at a football game having fun with her friends. I didn't have anyone at all.

By that evening, I could barely breathe. I called my mom, who told me to go to the hospital just to be safe. Somehow I drove myself there, only to find out there wasn't anything wrong with me. Nothing new, anyway. It was a minor panic attack, and I just needed to go home and rest and work through it.

At this point in my life, crying wasn't abnormal. The last time I'd really cried like that, though, was in the dark corner of my room just after being told I'd be dead in ten years. The breakup hit me hard. Maybe it was more difficult than the diagnosis. At least I had her to help me through that time. Now what was I supposed to do?

For a few months, I let the emotional hit of the breakup control me. I felt like I'd lost everything. I felt like I was worthless. I stopped working on my business. I almost gave up on keto. I stopped doing everything.

It took me a while to realize it, but I had relied on the relationship and not on myself. To get back on my feet, I had to reintroduce myself to...myself. Who was I? What was I capable of? Where did I want to go?

This new obstacle was huge. Yet another completely unexpected turn in my life. I could have hidden behind it and kept myself stuck. Or I could plow through it and find a new me just waiting to go after my dreams.

Change is going to happen. Change is going to *suck*. The thing is, I had no idea how much I needed that breakup. It took a long time. It took a lot of work getting to know myself. But I had relied on the relationship so much that if we hadn't broken up, I wouldn't be where I am today. I wouldn't be writing this book or growing my business. I wouldn't know what I really wanted out of life if I hadn't been forced to look inward and really figure myself out, apart from anyone else. So yeah, change is hard, but it's normal and it's not a bad thing. Don't let yourself get trapped in the emotions of it. Plow through and get to the other side!

DECISIONS

noun, plural. a conclusion or resolution reached after consideration.

synonyms: commitment, resolve, determination

Within months, I'd been diagnosed with brain cancer, had major surgery, completed weeks of chemo and radiation, lost and gained a business, become more or less a college failure, and lost the girl of my dreams. I didn't have friends, I stood out everywhere I went, and my doctors had told me I was on my deathbed.

What now?

It's human nature to want to wallow in sadness. When life keeps hitting us with setbacks and barriers, sometimes it's easier to just stop fighting. We feel sorry for ourselves, hoping that one day the difficulties will stop coming and *then* we'll be able to achieve our goals.

The only way out is forward, and that's what I had to decide for myself. I couldn't stand being in the college environment anymore, especially with my ex-girlfriend and I still in the same classes. That made the breakup that much harder to get over, and I never wanted a degree anyway. But I also wasn't ready to move to Austin on my own yet. I had to make a decision.

I knew what I wanted to do, but I was uneasy about making the decision because it didn't look like my grand plans of dropping out to run a thriving business from my dream apartment. Christmas break had just started, and driving home without my girlfriend was strange and depressing. Our families are practically neighbors, and a Christmas without her just highlighted how much things had gone wrong.

Fortunately, I had a great role model.

Just as my dad showed me what it was to keep looking for solutions even when everyone said they didn't exist, my mom showed me how to be decisive. When I told my mom I thought I might want to drop out, even though things weren't exactly perfect, she didn't hesitate. I think that, with everything I'd been through, she would have supported a decision to focus on my health, even without the business as a factor. But when we talked about how my business was doing and how much more I could focus on it, she made the decision seem easy. We drove back to campus and moved everything out of my dorm in a day and then never looked back. I had no one to say goodbye to. I had no reason to miss it. It was time to move on, and so I did.

I moved home with a new focus and fewer fears. I didn't have any reason to worry about "what ifs" for my business. There were no professors over my shoulder, taking up my time and telling me what I couldn't do. It was just me and this new life, and a big goal of moving downtown as soon as I could.

That's the great thing about rock bottom. There's nowhere to go but up. Mostly, anyway.

Moving back home opened a lot of doors for me and let me save money to reach my goals. I'm so grateful to my parents for being supportive of me, but moving home wasn't the biggest deal. It was the way they showed me how to face problems head on. They taught me to face my fear, shake its hand, and take back control of my life.

So many of us will sit around, day after day, trying to figure out what decisions we need to make. The worst casualty of that internal battle is *time*. We can never get that time back. The question isn't what decision you need to make. It's whether you're going to let fear steal more of your time. The unknown is scary. I get it. But you know what it is you want to do. Go with your gut. Make a decision. Change your life.

REFRAME

verb. to frame (something) again and often in a different way.

New diet, new lifestyle, new business, a new business partner who reached out to help me take things to the next level...heck, I could even think of my diagnosis as new. I had to think about everything differently in order to stay focused on my vision. When the doctors told me there was nothing I could do, I had the option to think about how many people have died from cancer and how insurmountable those odds were. I also had the ability to think about how incredible it was that I was in the low percentage of people who came out of surgery, took to treatments incredibly well, and was still healthy and doing well. I'd beaten the odds.

The same was true for my business. Nine out of ten

startups fail, so the professor had every right to tell me I was being unrealistic. It's one of the many negative perspectives we take as a society. *Treatment will make you miserable. It's too hard to write a book.* For every negative perspective we have—*I'll never be able to reach that goal*—there's a way to beat the odds. There's a way to reframe the fears and doubts to get to the other side. That way is simple: it's how you spend your time.

If you don't spend your time making good foods and working out, of course you won't lose weight. If you don't spend your time writing, of course you won't finish your book. Every minute of every day can get you closer to or further away from your goals. The way you spend that moment, from your mindset to your actions, is what makes the difference.

One negative message that I've had to overcome is one that's incredibly connected to how we spend our time. It's the idea that *social media is toxic.*

Just after I dropped out of college, when I was really focusing on building my business, all of my time went into social media. That's how I was building my business, so even though everyone said it was a waste of time and a negative influence, I had to do it. Then again, keto was brand new at the time, and talking about it brought a lot of unwanted attention. I got a ton of hate for it. It was so different than what everyone else was doing—too much fat for the bodybuilders, too much meat for the vegetarians—and there was not enough familiarity yet for people to really connect with it. The trolls showed up in full force, not just about how I was eating, but with personal attacks about me and my story.

I could have let that backlash confirm everyone's idea that it's a horrible waste of time to be involved in social media. But on the other side of that negativity, social media had become my connection to the world. Not only was I able to build my business, meet new people, and interact with them thanks to social media, but I also got in touch with experts.

From the beginning of my keto journey, I'd been hungry for more information. I kept looking up anything I could find about keto—diets, tips, meals, recipes—and Dr. Eric Berg would always pop up. He's a world-renowned doctor and keto pioneer, and I was and still am one of his three million subscribers. I watched everything he published.

At this point, I was really happy with how I was doing with keto. I felt like I was really going after it and seeing great results. One day though, I actually got Dr. Berg's attention on his live stream, and he answered my question while he was recording. I explained my diagnosis and how much I loved keto and how I hadn't fallen off the wagon, then I asked him what he would do in my shoes.

I really didn't think there was anything else I could do, but he immediately told me to go organic. All of the food I'd been eating was fine, except that quality made the difference. "If I were you, I wouldn't eat anything that's not organic."

I was so let down. Immediately my mind went to all of the reasons I couldn't do it. It would be too difficult, too expensive, too restrictive. One of my favorite things in the world was going out to eat with people, and now it was going to be almost impossible. And it was hard enough to keep friends as it was.

I had to reframe those thoughts, just as I'd done with the professor and the doctors, but this time for myself. I couldn't stop. I couldn't slow down. If this was the next step away from cancer, I had to take it. Instead of limiting my diet, I thought of it as upgrading my health and went out for all new groceries...again.

Time and mindset are really the keys—to almost anything. How you frame your mindset helps you spend your time, and how you spend your time determines whether or not you'll succeed. I was on social media for most of my day, but I spent that time investing in people and helping them with their goals. So did Dr. Berg, and that gave me the next step I'd needed to improve my health.

The people you follow and the messages you're around are going to influence your daily habits. By choosing negative voices, you're really influencing yourself. You're hanging on to the easy path of fear and excuses. Instead, follow people who are going to build you up. Invest in the right mindset and encouragement every day, so that whenever circumstances are outside of your control, you're ready to face them.

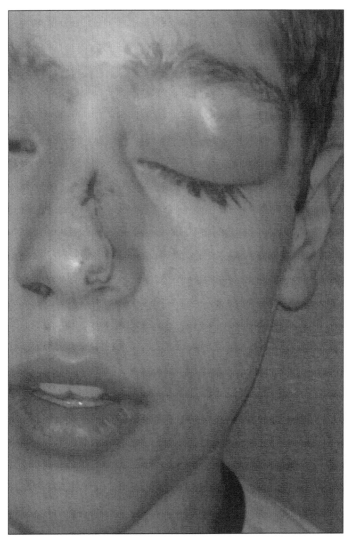

This was six years before the six-year-old tumor was removed. It happened in a basketball game—a traumatic injury straight to the skull, on the left side where the tumor was.

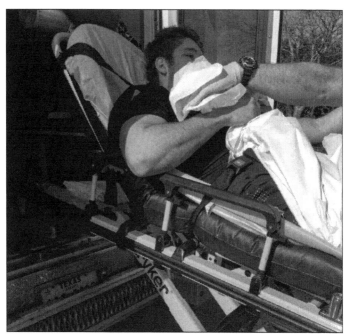

March 6, 2016. This is about thirty minutes after the car fell into the ditch. They broke into my car in order to get me out and transported me to the hospital.

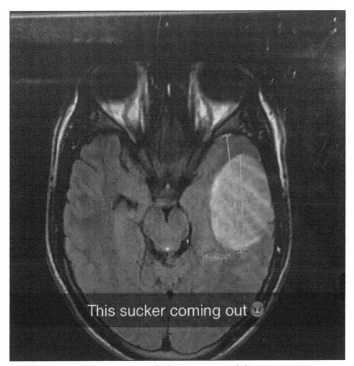

The MRI results of my brain tumor before surgery and diagnosis.

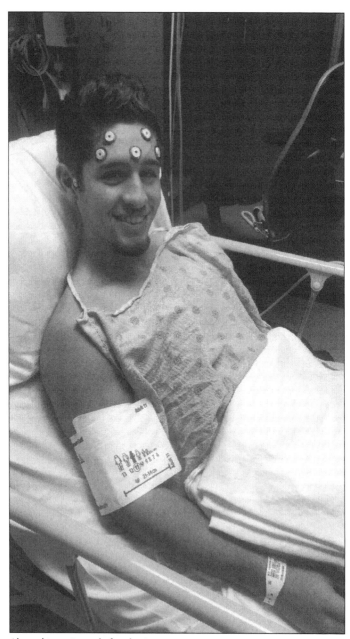

About thirty minutes before brain surgery.

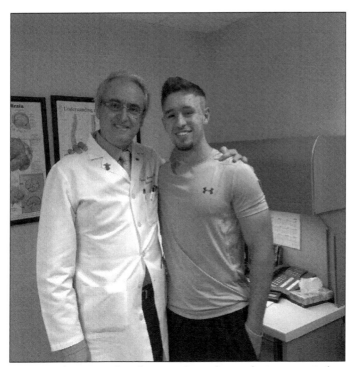

Dr. Raymond Sawaya, who is known as the number one brain surgeon in the world. He removed my tumor, 100 percent.

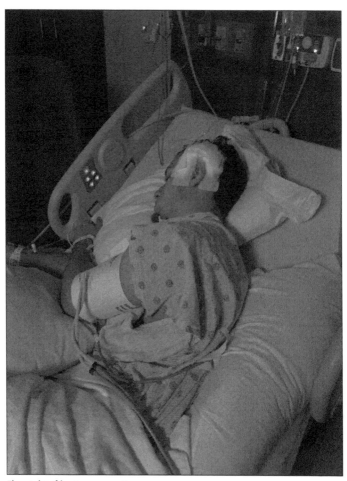

The night of brain surgery, in my recovery process.

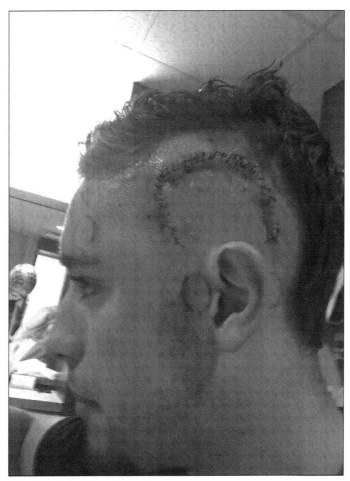

About two days after brain surgery.

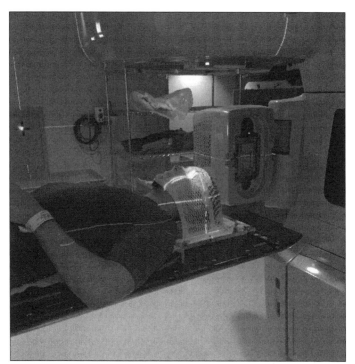

This was one of my first radiation sessions, which took place for about forty-five minutes every day.

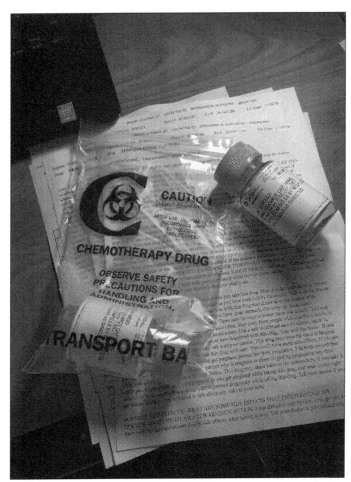

The chemotherapy capsules that I was given. I had to take these every day for over twelve weeks.

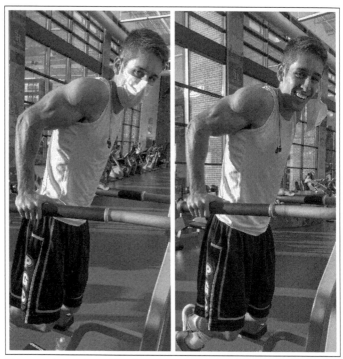

This was taken in the middle of my chemotherapy process—along with my goals to become leaner and healthier!

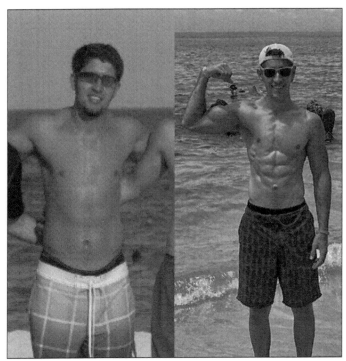

My ninety-day transformation through the ketogenic diet and my personal
FusionLean program.

HONORING YOUR SELF-WORTH

"Sometimes the hardest part of the journey is believing you're worthy of the trip."

—GLENN BECK, *THE CHRISTMAS SWEATER*

* * *

Early FusionLean

It's getting pretty tiring, how much hate I'm getting.

"How is that going to be sustainable?"

"Why are you forcing yourself into this diet?"

"You're torturing yourself!"

Maybe they're right...but I don't think I've forced myself into anything. Discipline isn't the same as being forced! This is what I've got to do to be healthy. To live.

I could skip the organics and eat out more, or I could stay alive. I could eat ice cream, or I could keep living. I don't think the choice is that hard, honestly. I feel great, and I'm another day closer to the cancer not coming back. So I guess they don't have to understand why I'm doing this. It's not their life on the line.

* * *

PERSPECTIVE

noun. a particular attitude toward or way of regarding something; a point of view.

synonyms: attitude, frame of mind, vantage point

I was only twenty years old, but I was learning some intense life lessons. After my diagnosis, I wanted and needed a miracle. The thing is, miracles come from action. They come from our thoughts. If you really need a miracle, you have to work at it.

The hard work mentality wasn't new for me. I've always worked at being an athlete and trying to become an entrepreneur. But that was before everything started falling apart. Now I had to work against the odds to get to where I wanted to be. I had to be active rather than passive.

When you have a passive mentality, you want things to just happen for you. You want to wait until everything is just right before you take action. You let the struggles pile up and you use them as an excuse to not move forward. Then we wonder why people fail, why they aren't happy, why they don't have money or aren't in shape. All that time lost in overthinking, looking for reasons not to act, and trying to decide what to do is holding us back.

Since the day of my seizure, my passive world had been challenged. It's like people are afraid to be hopeful, so they give you the worst-case scenario. Not only did I have to become active in pursuing my goals, but I had to actively change my thoughts too. When the doctor told me chemo would be horrible, I had to change my perspective from *this will suck* to *well, it's going to be difficult.* After the call with Dr. Berg, I walked into the kitchen and looked at everything I couldn't have. I had to change my perspective, from *starting over again* to *upgraded groceries means upgraded health.*

It's not normal to only eat organic food, much less only organic keto. But then again, it's not normal to defy the odds and beat brain cancer either. I had to change my perspective from *it'd be okay to live a little* to *you have to do this to stay alive.*

Every day, I made my own foods, focusing on quality and

organic sources. Then I'd share them on social media, alongside my progress and the progress people were sharing with me. They saw me enjoying my life, enjoying my food, and overcoming the odds. They saw how choosing different foods could give them the results they wanted. The hate didn't end—in fact, the bigger my platform became, the worse it got. But it couldn't stop me. I had a business to build and cancer to beat. I'd have to keep going in spite of their negativity.

There are no paths in this life that won't run into roadblocks. Eventually, you're going to face one. The bigger your goals, the more roadblocks you'll face. The only thing you can do is turn it into a reward. I didn't want to go all organic at first, but once I did, I was one step closer to my goals.

It's normal to want more than what we have or to wish we weren't facing hard times. But when we focus on that little bit that we wish were different, we often lose sight of the bigger picture. It's like the grass being greener on the other side of the fence—but a whole goldmine is behind you that you haven't even seen. Get a clear vision of what you're going after and let that fuel you to face the obstacles and negativity head-on. The life you're dreaming of is just on the other side.

16

SELF-WORTH

noun. confidence in one's own worth or abilities; self-respect.

synonyms: pride, dignity, morale, confidence, self-assurance, assurance

My whole life, I've always been determined to get better and better at everything I do. In middle school, I wanted to be a starter on my basketball team. In high school, I wanted to be the MVP. Nothing was going to stop me from reaching my goals, though for a while it felt like that came at a price.

Once, during basketball season, Coach Duffield showed me a video from a motivational speaker, and it made such an impact on me that I started watching something motivational every single day. Hearing their encouragement has always fueled me and kept me going.

Just then, at the beginning of my business and my life as a cancer survivor, some of those messages started to bring me down. I listened to speakers telling me to "bring value to the world," but the message that I heard was closer to, "If you're not bringing value to the world, you're not much of anything."

Without any friends to lean on, and a business partner who was increasingly unavailable, I looked to social media to tell me whether I was bringing value to the world. I wanted people to admire what I was doing and to give me that sense of approval. But because I was getting so much hate, that wasn't really meeting my need for validation. Either the doubters were just louder than the people seeing benefit, or there really were more of them. Either way, I wondered whether I was bringing something good to the world or just creating more chaos. My confidence dropped lower and lower, and I started to wonder whether I had any value to offer at all.

It wasn't actually their words hurting me, though. I was defeating myself. In my diet and my business, I was making massive leaps and seeing growth—but I wasn't growing as a person. We spend so much time thinking about being good enough for her, good enough for him, good enough to be liked, good enough to succeed, that we forget to be good enough for ourselves. Until we value ourselves first, it's always going to be a struggle to find that confidence and really feel like we're bringing value to the world.

I had kept my eyes on the vision, which helped me move forward in my business and health goals...but I hadn't really thought about myself. The journey isn't really about becoming an athlete or a millionaire or a coach. It's about becoming the best version of ourselves. Until I grew my own self-worth and understood who I was, I would always be pulled down by external voices telling me who they thought I was. A cancer patient, a hack, a loner, a dropout. The labels become a leash that drags us down and holds us back. The only way to counter them is to understand who we really are.

At twenty-one years old, I had what I needed to move to the Domain in downtown Austin. It didn't help my business or change my diet. It didn't get me closer to a doctor or a trainer. This was about meeting a goal I'd set years before, just for me. The real me, underneath the cancer and the keto and the social media presence.

This was a huge milestone for me. In spite of everything, I'd kept going and made enough money to move out. Finally, I could feel the accomplishment and do something just for myself. Moving day was incredible. My family helped me get everything into my apartment, and it all felt so exciting.

Then they gave me a hug, shut the door behind them...
and it was just me.

My actions said I valued myself—I ate well, did what I could to stop feeding the cancer, and prioritized my business. But internally, I was swayed by other people's opinions. Every time they questioned whether I was on the best path, whether my diet was sustainable, whether I needed to be on social media so much, I questioned myself too. If I kept doing that, I wouldn't be able to pursue my business or keep myself healthy.

I can't say it enough: we have to be our own biggest influencers. There are so many voices in our heads every day, so many outside standards we have to meet. If you're a person who has goals and dreams, those external objectives can completely take over. Our worth as humans isn't found in what we do or make or accomplish. It's in who we are. We have to figure that out first. It's the foundation of all the other work. Without it, we'll crumble at the smallest storm.

CONFIDENCE

noun. self-assurance arising from appreciation of one's own abilities or qualities.

synonyms: belief in oneself, positiveness, assertiveness, self-possession, nerve

Moving out was a huge motivator for me. It reminded me that the business was more than just social media, and that helped me start to approach it differently. I started to pay attention to the clients who were seeing results, which brought more people in who were curious rather than angry. They'd enroll, see results, and share their testimonials and before and after photos, then even more would visit to see what we were doing. The snowball effect had begun, and I felt better about deleting hateful comments as they came up rather than dwelling on them.

I had found confidence in myself, and now I was regaining confidence in what I was doing.

I wanted to be a fitness coach so I could bring value to people's lives and see them change their lives. Instead of focusing on the people trying to destroy that value, I saw the good that I was doing and started to enjoy it again.

One night, I made an Instagram post about my story and the dinner I was making, then sat down to listen to an episode of Andy Frisella's podcast, *The MFCEO Project*, while I ate. He talked about how people who are the most hateful are usually the ones who need the most help. They aren't where they want to be in their lives, so they try to take other people down with them. They want everyone else to be stuck like they are.

I thought back over the past few months living on my own. When my family had left to go back home that first day in my apartment, I realized just how alone I was. It hadn't gotten any better either. Working on my business had taken up most of my time, especially as my business partner seemed to see himself more as an advisor than an active partner. I'd hustle all week long without any complaints, working on my plans and site and mediating social media. Then on the weekends, when everyone else was out hanging out with people and having fun, it was still just me. I loved going out and being around people, but since I didn't have anyone, I just stayed in and kept working or went back to my family's house to spend time with them.

In other words, it was just me and my social media feed, for far too long. I would refresh for comments and watch as they came in, which means I saw almost every single hateful message. They weren't just negative either. They were mean. They blamed my plans for causing cancer. They told me I was making it all up just to make money. They told me they hoped I died. They told me they hoped I died *of cancer*.

If they were just trying to pull me down, it worked for a long time.

I would lie in bed reading comments until eleven or twelve, fall asleep, then wake up to do it all over again. Sometimes I would wake up in the middle of the night and check my phone to see if anyone else had commented. I was constantly reading, responding, and taking every little comment way too seriously.

That night after I finished dinner, I checked in on the post I'd made. The very first comment said, "You're such a scam artist. Stop posting this bullshit."

Then another one came in behind it: "You're right, bro. This is ridiculous."

Then another one: "Right? He's just making money off of cancer. This'll come back around to get him."

As I scrolled, my heart started to race. I could see myself getting ready for brain surgery, getting another blood draw, running another test. Sweat beaded up on my forehead and I could feel my chest tighten up.

All of that panic and anger boiled over into a response I typed up furiously. These dudes were about to see exactly how I felt about their doubts.

Before hitting send, I looked back at what I'd typed. I thought about Andy's episode that I'd just finished not an hour before. I thought about *How to Win Friends and Influence People* sitting on my nightstand. This wasn't killing with kindness. This wasn't empathy for the people spewing hate. This wasn't taking the high road. This wasn't what I was taught to do.

So I took a deep breath, deleted everything, and thought about why these people might want to drag me down to where they were.

I typed up a simple response:

> Hey, man. I appreciate you taking the time out of your day
> to express your thoughts. I'm not here to fight back, though.

I'm just here to learn from you guys in any way that I can. Thank you!

I took another deep breath and put my phone away for the night.

The next morning, I woke up to a message. It was from one of the people who had been so negative the night before. They said, "I want to apologize for me and my friends. I've actually looked up to you for some time now. If you're cool with it, I could use some help from you."

It was like a huge weight pulled off my back. Not every hater comes around like this. In fact, I usually just delete those comments as soon as they come in now, so that the rest of my followers can get the help they need. But it gave me the perspective I needed. I had something worthwhile to offer. People needed what I was sharing. And most of all, I needed to let go of the negativity in order to stay healthy.

Every time I let the angry comments create a negative reaction, I let them pull me down. I handed my confidence over. For all of the effort I put into eating healthy, I had let the doubts and anger take over. Maybe because I was afraid they were right. By getting defensive, I was giving them far too much control over my life.

It's okay to not have all the right answers. Stay open-minded and view challenges as an opportunity to grow if you need to—even if growth looks like hitting delete or letting go of the need for someone else's approval. Focus on what you can do, what you're driven to do, and what you will do—eliminate the doubts and what you can't do—and you'll step into real confidence that can't be shaken.

COMMITMENT

noun. being dedicated to a cause.

synonyms: dedication, devotion, adherence, loyalty

Brain cancer had brought destruction with it, a complete undoing of everything that I'd been comfortable with in my life. But it also set me on a journey to become the best version of myself. The problem with that journey is there's not a finish line. There's always something more you can do, some other way you can grow. Ironically, when we keep going we become more confident, even though we never get to a point where we've "arrived." Confidence doesn't show up after doing something once or twice. It's a product of consistency—little actions that add up over time.

I saw this the most in my diet. Although I didn't cheat on my diet, I was constantly pressured to. People would tell me how I needed a cheat meal to live. They'd say the diet would affect my mental health if I didn't break it now and then. And honestly? I'd never seen anyone as committed to keto as I was. I didn't know if they were right, because I had no one to compare my life to. Since my doctors weren't directing my diet, they couldn't help either.

Looking at my internal standards, I didn't think I was wrong. All of my MRI follow-ups came back with great results. My social media presence was growing—in supporters now, not haters. My business was thriving. I was reading all kinds of encouraging books. I was happy with my body and not chasing diet fads or trying to bulk up/ lean out over and over every time the season changed. I felt really good about my life. I approved of myself, no matter what anyone else thought, and that gave me a lot of confidence to stay so committed to my diet.

Still, I wanted to keep learning. I wanted to know if they were right. Was a cheat meal really important?

There's a nutritionist here in Austin who has a waitlist of almost a year long. Because my situation is so precarious, I was able to get in with him sooner. I told him everything I was doing and asked him what else there was to know.

Our conversation was so encouraging. He affirmed every-thing I was doing, then offered a list of supplements that he thought might help. I'm always hungry for something proactive that I can do, and he fueled me up. Then he told me something amazing:

If you keep doing what you're doing, and you really commit to it, this isn't going to come back.

The doctors who said there was nothing to do had no hope and no instructions for me. This doctor, who was just as world-renowned as the others, had a completely different perspective. He was proud of the work I was doing and so excited to see my results. I knew he would know about cheat meals, too, so I asked him if everyone was right. Did I need to cheat a little in order to be a whole human being?

He told me that, with the way my body adapted to the diet, a cheat meal would probably make me feel miserable, but it wouldn't actually hurt me.

Literally everyone was telling me a slice of pizza wouldn't hurt, but was that really true? My perspective shifted again. Even if it wasn't guaranteed to bring my cancer back or anything dramatic, what if that one slice made me feel horrible and then took more work to get back on track? Even worse, what if that one slice spiked my blood sugar just enough to spark the cancer cells again and let them take root? If my cancer ever came back, would I want that one slice of pizza hanging over my head, making me wonder if I could have done anything to avoid it?

On yet another level, was it worth letting the comments and questions take root in my mindset?

I absolutely loved the foods I could eat. I loved the life I was building. There was no reason to break my commitment. I was onto something, and I wanted to see how far I could take it.

It's so natural to want other people to approve of us. In high school, I always wanted to have tons of friends, good hair, and cool clothes. It still feels good to have people like me and approve of what I'm doing. But if you're not happy with yourself, if you don't value yourself, how can other people value you? Real confidence comes before outside approval, not after.

To build up your confidence, you have to stay committed. They're connected, a million times over. Think about the first time you went to the gym. You probably felt more apprehension than confidence. But if you go again, then go again, and then start to see results, and build it into your routine. Eventually the commitment you build up creates confidence. And the more you value yourself, the easier it is to commit.

PATIENCE

noun. the capacity to accept or tolerate delay, trouble, or suffering without getting angry or upset.

We all want things to happen right *now*. We want the success, the change, the results. That's why supplements are top-selling products. People buy supplements before meal plans and workouts because they're hoping it'll be the easy route.

I'm not any different. Patience is one of my biggest weaknesses, and I'm still working on it. I wanted immediate success in my business and I've always wanted immediate changes in my body. I even wanted the cancer to be immediately gone after surgery.

Even if we don't get immediate results, we want immediate answers. Will the keto diet take care of my body? Will my business be sustainable? That's why social media can be such a dangerous place—it gives us the immediate feedback that we think we need. If we don't get that validation, we start to question ourselves. We crave instant gratification, and it's hard to learn to be patient.

In my constant search for ways to starve cancer, I learned about intermittent fasting. Talk about learning to let go! There was so much information about it. I read about how it stimulates natural human growth hormone, how much it helps men especially, and how it could build on the keto diet to take cancer starvation to the next level. It felt like discovering keto all over again. I was so excited to get started.

As Americans, what gives us more instant gratification than food? We think about eating all the time, and if we want something we go get it. It's odd to go sixteen, eighteen, twenty hours a day without eating. The first morning I tried to fast, I got up as usual and answered some emails. Then I walked into the kitchen to make breakfast, the same way I had my entire life. I had to stop myself. At first my fast was to stop eating at 8 p.m. then skip breakfast, and even that felt odd.

Fasting was definitely not the norm for my audience or peers either. I was told I was starving myself, that I would lose muscle. Just like when I'd started keto, people lashed out against this thing that was completely unfamiliar to them.

Then the time came for another MRI and a visit with my neuro-oncologist. The test came back clear, as always, and we talked about how I was feeling. I didn't have any headaches or slurred speech; everything seemed fine. And I was excited to tell him about intermittent fasting. I thought he would be excited about the research I had done and that I was being proactive. Instead, he shrugged me off.

"That may not work for everyone, but it's worth a try."

Great. Another doctor writing me off. Why can't my doctors have even a little bit of faith in what I'm doing? A little bit of hope that the odds might be wrong?

I could feel myself slipping back into anger and depression again, and I had to remind myself that their lack of faith didn't have to become my own. I didn't need their support. I didn't need anyone's approval. I didn't need to know right now whether it was going to keep my cancer at bay. I could learn to be patient and do what I knew was right for me.

It wasn't easy to break the instant gratification habits that

I'd lived with for so long. I thought more about breaking my fast than I ever did about having a cheat meal. But after a while, I settled in and grew to enjoy it.

For me, intermittent fasting looked like two meals a day starting at 2 p.m., plus a little bit of a fat snack in between. Eventually, I stretched it out into one big meal and one snack. I eat everything I would have before, but I give my body most of the day to process it instead of eating nonstop. My meals are amazing, with loads of asparagus, spinach, broccolini, eggs, salmon, grass-fed steaks, nuts, and rich oils. I love what I'm eating and I feel great about when I eat. Most of all, I'm learning to be patient and to take care of myself even when the rest of the world asks me to indulge.

To unlock your own greatness, you have to be patient with the process. Little decisions lead to big growth, but only if you can stick with them. You might have a mountain in front of you, but that doesn't mean you have to scale it all at once. Keep taking those little steps, let the results come when they will, and you'll get there. The amazing thing is, when you're taking little steps in your mindset, in your habits, in your belief, and in your confidence, it all adds up. One day you'll look back and see just how far you've come.

MOTIVATION

noun. the reason or reasons one has for acting or behaving in a particular way.

synonyms: incentive, stimulus, inspiration, incitement.

I loved seeing my business grow. People's lives were changing. Where at first no one knew about keto, it was picking up in popularity. I spent a ton of time creating content, growing my brand, and becoming a public figure.

Since childhood, I had wanted to secure my financial freedom. My parents were always supportive. They told me to do whatever would make me happy, and they were clear that money wouldn't be the answer. Freedom to me looked like working for myself. I grew up on social media and imagined how cool it would be to live the life of an influencer. They seemed to be able to do whatever they wanted, whenever they wanted. That's the life that I had in mind.

But the bigger it grew, the more there was to do, and I was completely alone. Not only was I alone without friends to hang out with in real life, but I was alone in my business. My partner, Ron, had come on board early on with the goal of helping me grow my business. I gave him part ownership and was excited to see how far we could take it. After months of working together, though, it was clear that we had different ideas about what that meant. We met up at the beginning of the year and talked big picture, then he more or less disappeared. I was left to do all the legwork while he traveled and focused on his other ventures.

I'd made enough money to live on my own, but I hadn't secured any freedom. I felt tied down to the business and was increasingly frustrated that it all fell on me. At first, I thought he was only gone for that one trip. Then he'd go out of the country for weeks at a time. When he was home, there was no time for us to get together because he had the next thing to get ready for. I felt trapped.

First thing in the morning, I would wake up and start tackling comments. Then I'd wade through emails before trying things to grow the business. Before I knew it, I was working until I crashed and then waking up to do it all over again. My energy started to slip and stress started to grow. I started to wonder if running the business was my dream life after all.

Then a client reached out with some feedback. His name was Danny Florea, and he had come to me twelve weeks before, asking what he could do to look like me. He was serious about it—ready to change his life. I'd watched him work the plans and stay more dedicated than anyone ever had. At the end of those twelve weeks, he sent a before and after with the comment, "You have changed my life."

I was shocked. This was the most inspiring transformation I had ever seen. Not only had he lost the significant amount of weight that he was originally worried about, but he had grown as a person. He had new routines, new habits, and more confidence.

He reminded me why I was building this business in the first place.

I reached out to my business partner and told him what was going on. I explained how dangerous stress was for my body—for my brain—and told him I couldn't do it anymore. I couldn't let the business turn into a risk to my health, and I didn't want to lose sight of what I was after.

To his credit, he respected what I had to say. My health was too important. My goals for the business were too important. That's what it really came down to—we partnered up but hadn't made sure our goals were aligned. He knew fitness and he knew business, but he wasn't in it as a partnership. He thought of it more like an investment and expected to just oversee, check in, and do some high-level thinking. He was in it for the check, and I was in it for the direct influence.

After we parted ways, a follower of mine named Garvan Smyth started checking in to see if he could help. Off and on for about six months, Garvan would put work in to help me out, asking if we could work together. Eventually, I could tell that we were working toward the same goals. We were becoming friends and worked well together. He wanted to bring value to the business, not to me, because he believed in what we were doing.

That's what I had needed in a partner—someone motivated by the same things I was. Now we stay in touch every single day, share the workload, and enjoy both our own freedom and the results we bring to our followers. That's what I had needed to make my business more sustainable.

By understanding what really motivated me toward this vision, I was able to see where the business didn't align. We think we know our whys and what makes us do certain things, but how often do we really evaluate this? Why are you at this point in your life? Why are you headed in this direction? Every now and then, take a step back to see where you are, where you're going, and why. You might be surprised at what you find.

LIMITS

noun. a restriction on the size or amount of something permissible or possible.

There's a cycle to the fitness world. In the winter, it's bulk season. Everyone's worried about getting swole. In the summer, it's shred season. Time to get ready for the beach. For years, I went with the patterns. I followed everybody else. It affected the calories I ate and the way I worked out. Now I couldn't let those things drive me.

The cancer was my number one priority, which meant my eating stayed stable all year long. Over the two years that had passed since the seizure, that morning when I was ready for summer shredding, my body dropped into a new normal all its own. I dropped from just over 200 pounds to 145, then stabilized naturally there. I stayed lean and felt good in my body without worrying about keeping up with anyone else.

Without constantly trying to perfect my body, I was free to work on my mind.

I started with my sleep, building on habits that started back when I let go of my reliance on social media. Instead of checking comments in the middle of the night, I put my phone in another room entirely. I learned that Wi-Fi and electronics around my head could be interrupting my sleep, and that sleep could affect whether or not the tumor came back. I learned that sleep affects stress and anxiety, emotions, and mental strength. When I put all of the factors together—my body, my energy, my mind, my cancer—I knew that sleep had to be the first thing I fixed. As soon as I made it a priority, my morning energy changed completely.

Next, I worked on a morning routine. My good friend Hal Elrod wrote an incredible book called *The Miracle Morning*, and it inspired me to be more intentional about my day. The first thing I thought about was getting my mindset right instead of rolling over and pulling the covers back up. So I started my days by turning on a motivational video and doing one hundred push-ups. My mind had to grow more than my body for that to work, but I made it a priority. By getting started as soon as I got up, the battle for my morning was already won.

Before, I had just wanted to work out. I never prioritized stretching. When I learned about how tightness can lead to inflammation, stress, and lower productivity, it became the next piece to build into my morning routine. Once the push-ups were done, I started to stretch. I worked on improving blood flow, releasing tightness, and increasing physical performance.

With my body and mind awake, I sit down to read a book for about an hour. The books I choose can all solve a problem or inspire some kind of personal improvement—Hal Elrod, Grant Cardone, Gary V...I look for the most successful people in the world and then follow what they've done to get there. My phone stays off and in another room, because I'm not quite done restoring my mind and body for the day ahead. Each of these steps is as important as sleep. By reading first thing in the morning, I fill my mind with positive thoughts about what I can accomplish and how I need to focus my day. After that, I pull out my journal and rewrite my life goals, because writing inspires belief. Then I write about the amazing day ahead, setting intentions that will carry me the rest of the day.

We don't have control over what's coming each day, but we can keep our minds focused as we face them. So I finish my day with some deep breathing and meditation. It's not something rigid or frustrating. It's just time that I take before the day starts. I get comfortable on the couch and take some deep breaths in and out, picturing them cleansing me internally and externally. I visualize all of my goals being achieved. I picture what it will be like to speak to people all around the world. I picture my book in my hands. I picture what it will take to make those goals a reality. I remember how much my mind has been capable of and how much more it can do.

How you start your day is usually how you end your day. Getting my morning under control got my whole day under control. I noticed a difference in my days right away. After one great day, then another, and another, my new routine quickly became a habit. It's not even a second thought anymore. It's just how I start my day.

Once you begin to prioritize your mental and emotional health as much as your physical health, everything else changes as well. You begin to level up as a person. You boost your self-worth, confidence, and peace with yourself and your day. Taking time to yourself in the morning teaches you how to be alone, how to be okay with who you are. You learn how to break out of that feeling of being trapped and stuck and how to find real, internal, limitless freedom.

CONNECTION

"A dream you dream alone is only a dream. A dream you dream together is reality."

—JOHN LENNON

* * *

Two Years Post-Diagnosis

For my twenty-first birthday, we found a high-quality restaurant where I could actually eat. I decided to get a single glass of wine, since wine is the most keto-friendly alcohol. It was such a great time, it reminded me how much I love hanging out with people.

It's time to bring people back into my life. I've invested so much into my business and my health, but I haven't reached out beyond social media in a very long time. Honestly, I'm scared to death. I'm a social media influencer, which is decently hard to find. I'm twenty-one. Also hard to find, off campus anyway. Oh, and I'm a brain cancer patient who only eats keto inside a four-hour window every day. That's not exactly normal. Will I find anything in common with anyone?

Who's going to want to bring a brain cancer patient into their life anyway?

* * *

DISCOMFORT

noun. a state of unease, worry, or embarrassment.

When I was first diagnosed, I was up for anything. I was grabbing at straws, hoping to find something that would help even a little bit. My life was on the line. What I ultimately learned is that winning isn't about just surviving. It's about focusing on every facet of your life. It's beyond your health, beyond your diet, beyond the one goal you have right now. If you want to beat something like brain cancer, you have to work on absolutely everything, from your mindset to your relationships to the control you have over yourself and your day. You have to become your own CEO. You have to get uncomfortable.

The more I grew, the more I learned. I was hungry for information that could help me get a little closer to complete health—and that has become a constant process. There's no room for short bursts of "I'm ready!" then falling off after a week goes by. I have to dig deep to find constant motivation.

At first, I thought I could get that motivation from the outside. I looked to doctors and experts, only to be disappointed. I wanted motivation from my professor but instead got shut down. I relied on my girlfriend for encouragement and wound up losing the woman I thought I would marry.

Once I realized the motivation had to come from within, things changed. I let go of that need for approval and started embracing all of the steps I knew I had to take, big and small. I leaned into keto. I learned how to fast. I learned about cell phones and shampoo and water. And I never stopped learning. I learned that the scratched up pans I'd been cooking in or the plasticware I'd been serving my food on could be a problem, so I invested in new cookware and plates and silverware. I leveled up from putting my phone out of my bedroom at night to taking all my calls from earbuds or over the speaker. I took supplements, met with nutritionists, listened to new doctors, and learned what each new thing could do to help prevent tumor regrowth.

Instead of being frustrated now when I learn that something needs to change, I think of it as a reward. It's another thing I've unlocked that can help me get closer to winning.

The more internal freedom I found, the more I wanted to face my fears and discomfort and anything left that was holding me back. The one thing left that I hadn't been able to heal? I still didn't have any friends. I needed to connect with people outside of social media...which had been easier said than done. So much so that I had put it off for years. But if there was one message all the speakers and authors kept telling me, it was to get comfortable being uncomfortable.

It was time.

I'd chosen my apartment in Austin because I thought it'd help me connect with new friends, especially older, more experienced people who I could learn from. There were plenty of people around who I could make friends with, if I could just get out there and do it. So I did.

I started going to coffee shops, looking for opportunities to talk to people. At a Starbucks nearby, I ran into a videographer that I knew, and he was talking to a girl I didn't know. I introduced myself to her and found out her name was Jamie and that she and her brother own a supplement company at the Domain, where I live. We're still good friends.

Once I broke the ice and started meeting people, I gained more confidence, and it all started to snowball. I found out I wasn't so alone after all. There are people who value their health just as much as I do, and my life or death situation doesn't change that much. We have similar approaches. We're all just trying to create the best version of ourselves.

The walls I put up around myself after the diagnosis weren't much different than the walls I'd always kept. Growing up, I was used to getting comfortable being uncomfortable, as long as it was physical. I worked out every day of the week, sometimes several workouts in a day. I took pride in my ability to stretch myself physically. But when it came to social and emotional discomfort, I held back. I wanted to make everyone happy and comfortable. I wanted them to like me. Eventually, I couldn't level up my life anymore if I stayed lonely and cut off from other people.

Once I was able to make new friends, I was ready to face anything. Improving my life has become a game, and I love playing it. By seeking discomfort out, intentionally looking for ways to stretch and grow, every day brings new wins. Every day gets me closer to knowing myself more and continuing to grow. Every challenge is something to be celebrated, even when it's unexpected, unfamiliar, or just plain scary.

I'll never forget meeting with a neuro-oncologist early on, Dr. Conrad, who told me about turmeric as an anti-inflammatory. It was an excellent appointment. He reminded me of that second neurosurgeon—so full of contagious confidence. He told me, "My job is to figure out how we can work around this disease for you. Your job is to do what I'm telling you to do and to enjoy life." I got an immediate boost of confidence from my connection with him...and the very next day, he died.

We're not on this journey alone, and we don't know how long the people around us will be here. Reach out to someone. Break up with loneliness. Find the thing that makes you uncomfortable and do it. Then do the next thing. Shake fear's hand and then move forward in spite of it. Move forward with good friends, good teachers, and good inspiration by your side.

DOUBT

noun. a feeling of uncertainty or lack of conviction.

synonyms: uncertainty, suspicion, confusion

Right after treatment, I went in for MRIs pretty fre-quently—every month or two. Glioblastoma doesn't migrate out into other parts of the body the same way other stage IV cancers do, but it can come back quickly and without much warning. There are some symptoms that I know to watch for, but the only way to know what's really happening in there is to take a look.

It didn't take long for MRIs to feel like routine tests, but I still dreaded the appointments. Not because of the pro-cedure, but because of the way the doctors treated me. They never had any solid answers and it almost felt like they were trying to get it to come back. I guess they were always trying to protect themselves, but it was nerve-wracking and frustrating, especially early on.

Early on, every time a doctor would shrug and write me off when I told them what I was doing, it cast doubt on all of my efforts. For a little while, doubt had started to control me. I was constantly second-guessing and looking for approval. The thing is, approval and validation are shifty. The first surgeon was sure that the surgery would go badly, but he was also sure that the tumor wasn't at a stage IV yet. The second surgeon was confident about the process, and then the diagnosis was a definitive stage IV.

There's a book on my shelf by Brendon Burchard called *Motivation Manifesto*, and on the cover it says, "Conformity is the jailer of freedom and the enemy of growth." Over time, I could look back at all of those moments where the experts were wrong or contradicted each other, and when I'd tried so hard to get them to approve of what I was doing. I realized that everyone has a different perspective and opinion, and I'll never be able to make them all happy or align with all of them at once. Slowly, I began to let them all go. I let go of my need for answers and clear outcomes. By working toward my goals no matter what, I began to let go of doubt—really, it let go of me.

Instead of looking for opinions, thoughts, and words to

affirm what I'm doing, I look for action. What can I do to learn and grow from this obstacle that I've been given?

A year or so into this whole journey, a company contacted me to see if I wanted to do their DNA test and then promote it on my platform. It seemed like a great opportunity to find out what might have led to the tumor, so I told them I'd do it. I got the packet in the mail, put a test strip under my tongue, then sent it back in for evaluation.

About a week later, thirty pages of information about my DNA sat in my inbox, and not one of them said cancer would be a problem.

On the other hand, I did learn a lot about myself that has nothing to do with the tumor. I learned that I tolerate caffeine and alcohol well, and that my heart and cognitive function are both in great shape. I could see nutrients that I was likely to be deficient in, and was happy to know that I already took the supplement that would fix it.

The most interesting thing I learned from that test was that I might have a tendency toward food addiction. It said that I could eat a lot without feeling full. That my mind and body want to operate on two different levels instead of working together.

As I read, I thought back to when I would eat 3,500 calories a day, or how I had no problem gaining or losing weight. I thought about how it took time to settle into intermittent fasting because I thought about food so much in the morning. I thought about how I could eat a lion's share of a meal and still want more, or how I still think about food around lunchtime when everyone else is grabbing tacos and I'm still waiting.

And then I thought about how all of those things might have fed—and could still feed—tumors.

If I were still looking for validation and justification from experts, that piece of information could have sent me into a tailspin. You can't fix your DNA, after all. It would have been an easy excuse to stop making hard choices and to give myself a break. Live a little, right? I could have taken any of the doctors' attitudes and used them as a reason to go easy on myself.

When you're going after something that you haven't done before, self-doubt has easy access. No one who has achieved great things let doubt hold them back. It's not that they never listened to limitations or questioned themselves—but they didn't stop because of it. To achieve uncommon results, you have to take uncommon actions.

I've taken an uncommon path, but then again, my situation isn't normal. There's no documented reason why

I got brain cancer. There's no way of knowing whether my unhealthy lifestyle made it happen, or if it was just a gift to help me grow. I don't know if I would eat the same way, have the same business, or enjoy the same internal growth that I have now if it weren't for cancer. I do know that, after overcoming so many obstacles and beating so many odds, action will always win over doubt, and doubt will always try to keep you from it. Don't stop. Don't worry. Don't doubt. Just take that ticket for a new opportunity and go.

At the end of the day, nothing can beat me besides me—not cancer, not breakups, not school, not fear, not doubt...not even my DNA. All of the things I've learned have come from experience, not from experts. The choices I made weren't guaranteed to help, but doing nothing was guaranteed to kill me. A lot of times it feels like taking a risk, but there's no downside. At the very least, you are going to learn something. If you let doubt hold you back, you'll never learn, you'll never grow, and you'll never know what could have been possible.

FIGHT

verb. move forward with difficulty, especially by pushing through.

One of the most dangerous things for a cancer patient—or anyone, for that matter—is stress. It feeds on doubt and creates overthinking. It kills confidence, recovery, and sleep. Stress also comes with a lot of inflammation, which triggers diseases all throughout the body. Diseases including cancer.

When my business felt like it was tying me down, that stress could literally have killed me. I had to take it seriously enough to consider whether the business was worth it. I can't let stress take hold in my life.

Then again, I'd been stressed from elementary school

when I worried about having great hair and getting the girls to like me. I'd sought perfection for my entire life, without ever rewarding myself or enjoying my accomplishments. I thought about the past, worried about the future, and never enjoyed the present moment.

Not only is stress bad for our health, but it's terrible for our mindset. It can keep us stagnant and block us from growth. It can hold us back from the future we want to create. It sets the tone for our days and takes over our lives. The sheer stress of watching for symptoms or waiting for a seizure could completely consume me. Since I can't really control tumors or what's happening inside my body, what good would that do? On the other hand, I *can* learn what might contribute to tumor regrowth and choose to take action.

Now, instead of reacting to stress by trying to ignore the problem, or even ignoring the stress itself, I use it as a gauge. If I'm feeling stressed, there's probably an opportunity for action. I think about what it is that has me stressed, then decide whether or not it's something I can control.

I can't control what doctors will tell me. I can't control what business partners will do. I can't control the way people will receive me. I can't control the cancer. But there is so much that is within my reach. I still have my choices, my diet, my mentality, my habits, my beliefs, my boundaries...Most of the time, focusing on what I can do alleviates some of the stress around what I can't do. It turns that stress into fuel and gets me back on the path toward my goals.

When we talk about cancer, we usually say that we're fighting it. It's an active word, and a lot of action is necessary. At the same time, you also have to learn to rest. To be patient. To breathe and accept the obstacle in front of you. We only exist in this moment. Whether you need to rest and be patient or take an action, stress can't hold you hostage when you let go of fear for the future or anxiety over the past.

I don't know yet if it's really possible to beat brain cancer, but if I stress about it, I'll never know. We don't beat stress by knowing what will happen in the future. This is just as true for starting a business, getting in shape, going after a job, or pursuing a tough degree. If you give in to stress, you'll never know what's possible. Accept your obstacles, face your fears, and conquer doubt, one step at a time.

FUTURE

noun. what will happen in the time to come.

Two years after my diagnosis, I had hit my stride. I had a
stack of clean MRIs behind me. My business was thriving.
My diet was still amazing. I had great friends, still lived
in a great location, and tackled every day with energy
and confidence. The more great results I got, the stronger my drive was to stay on the uncommon path. My fast
extended to twenty or twenty-two hours, with one giant
meal and a snack every day. When people told me I was
starving myself, I confidently responded that I was only
starving cancer.

I felt like I had a handle on my stress, my self-doubt, and
my self-limitations, which had been such a struggle in
the months before. Still, I never want to stop learning

and growing. I got on a waiting list to speak with a world-renowned doctor and expert on the keto diet. I didn't really have any complaints or specific things to ask him about, but I'm always trying to check in with experts to see what I can learn.

When I got through to him, he had great input. There were still household items I could replace, like laundry detergent and toothpaste, and it was all really helpful.

But that reminded me to tell him, and my parents, who were also on the line, that I did have a tooth that was scheduled for a root canal. It had been hurting for a couple of weeks and was starting to turn gray. It was gross and annoying and I was ready to get the procedure done so it would feel better.

The tone of the call immediately shifted.

After a pause, the doctor said, "Oh my God, you are kidding me."

I started sweating, thinking about what might come next as he went on to explain that the tooth dying was a sign of the tumor returning. He said I shouldn't go get the root canal, that I should go get an MRI first and take care of the tumor before anything else. This was a horrible sign and we needed to act right away. It would probably be more aggressive than before. It was not a good sign.

This wasn't the first time I'd been told over the phone that I was going to die, but you don't get used to it. It was a punch to the gut.

You do learn, however, to verify the details before you get worried. I called up a fellow brain cancer survivor, Greg Cantwell, who has outlived his tumor by fourteen years and counting. I explained the call to him and asked what he thought: "Have you ever heard of a toothache being a sign of a tumor?"

"No," he said, "I've worked with the top neuro-oncologists in the world, and I've never heard of that."

I was with him, for sure—this didn't sound right at all. But unlike my younger self, I wasn't just looking for validation. I wanted to know for sure, and now I had two different opinions to choose from.

I decided not to listen to either of them, really. Neither of them could know.

Instead, I listened to my gut. I thought about the signs we knew were connected to a tumor—weakness, fatigue, headaches, blurred vision, etc.—and checked in with how I'd been feeling. I did research on my own, just like I had with keto and fasting. I got my tooth fixed. And I waited.

About a month later, my routine MRI came back clean. No one knew what that was about, no one had heard of that as a sign. My instincts had been right, and I hadn't lost a month to stress or worry.

> The more work I put into my mental and emotional health, the easier it has been to take care of my physical health. It's helped me find joy and continually expand what's possible. That brief scare reminded me that I'm my own CEO.
>
> No one in your life should control you, except you. No one else can unless you let them. The steps you take every day to take back control are the steps that will help you conquer the odds. For me, that means beating cancer. It means proving my professor wrong and living out my dream of entrepreneurship. What will you do as the CEO of your own life?

26

URGENCY

noun. importance requiring swift action; an earnest and persistent quality; insistence.

I love talking to my customers, followers, and listeners about the things they're up against. I love it because I know what's possible. The thing that seems fully impossible now will look completely different once they've conquered it. Usually it's a goal they've been working on for a long time, or a sudden obstacle that they aren't sure how to get past. Most of the time, they know what they need to do. The problem is, it's way too easy for them to talk themselves out of taking action in the first place.

I don't know where I would be right now if I hadn't been diagnosed with cancer. I don't know what would have motivated me to grow up so much, so quickly—and I still have a long way to go. But I do know that the urgency that came with that diagnosis changed everything.

I didn't have a choice. There was no magic cure-all to wait for, no rescue coming. The odds are not in my favor to this day. If I don't push forward, every single day, I could lose time. I could die.

While I wouldn't wish my journey on anyone else, it might be a good mental exercise. If you put that same urgency into your own life, what would change? Cancer is a continual gun to my head, and the trigger could be pulled at any moment. What if you knew you had thirty days to make that habit? Six months to get your business off the ground? What if you had to change your eating habits or you would die?

If you live with the knowledge that time is valuable and we only have so much of it, it's harder to justify wallowing in self-pity. It's harder to give some of that time over to doubt and loneliness. You still can...but why would you?

When I was a kid, all of the influences and motivational icons in my life talked about time. I was able to catch enough of their meaning to develop a work ethic, but I never really understood the significance of time. For most of us, it isn't until something tragic happens that we find that urgency and the value of time.

Think about it. If you break a bone, you don't finish watching a show before you go to the ER. That natural urgency shifts our focus onto solving the problem.

So why is it that we don't have time to go to the gym, or we don't have time to work on the business we've dreamed about? Why don't we have time for ourselves, time in our mornings, time to sleep well? Do we have time for our kids, time for our friends, time for our family?

People who use the gift of time to their advantage don't wait for an emergency. They don't have to have a gun to their head or a diagnosis to overcome. None of us knows when we're going to die. Not even the most skilled doctor with a clear diagnosis knows who will beat the odds. Life is precious and can be taken away in an instant. These people know how precious time is, and they don't waste it.

Since knowing that I had to act quickly or my time might be up, I've been able to take risks. I've been able to experiment. I've been able to get uncomfortable and ultimately achieve my goals.

Now I act like cancer's coming for every aspect of my life. With the way I eat and take care of myself, I'm constantly reminded that consistency will save my life. Now I think about my business in the same way: what if not making

$2,000 on that new venture this month would bring the cancer back? What am I going to do to accomplish it then?

This isn't about losing yourself in your work. It's not about adding more stress, like *Logan said if I don't lose weight I'll die!* That's not it. Really, I just want to unlock your true capabilities. What is possible for you if you let go of your doubts, invest your precious time, and focus all of your energy and efforts on your goals?

What are you unhappy with? What do you want to create? What do you dream of?

The clock is ticking.

Remember this: there is no failure if you try. If you don't take the risk, you'll stay stuck in that job, at that weight, with that illness, with those unfulfilled dreams...but if you do try, if you do take action, you can't lose. No matter what, you'll learn something, and that's a huge win. Make the most of your time. Pick a course of action and get consistent with it. Get lots of input from different people. Do research. Experiment. Change your mindset.

Do the work now, before it's too late.

We don't have time to be passive. We don't have time to wait for everything to be perfect. Figure out what odds you're beating—accept the obstacle in front of you—and put that lens of urgency on your own life. What do you need to do to beat those odds? What will it take to achieve your dreams?

The moment you open your eyes to what's possible, even though there are obstacles in front of you, is the moment your journey begins. That's when the true beauty of life begins to unfold—when you know just how short it is and just how much you can accomplish in that time.

IMPOSSIBLE

adjective. not able to occur, exist, or be done.

antonyms: possible, easy, attainable.

Greg Cantwell, the first person I called to verify the doctor's fear about my tooth, is a fellow stage IV glioblastoma survivor. He travels around supporting and consulting people like me who feel alone in their diagnosis and journey. My mom found him early on, and we met up at a Starbucks in Kyle, Texas.

I poured my heart out to him that day. I told him everything I could possibly tell him about the doctors, the process, how I was feeling, and what I was worried about. He told me, "Look, I've been there. I know what it's like to have people tell you what's going to happen and what you should think. But you have to understand, you can't just base your beliefs on what one person is saying. You have to take action. You have to experiment. You have to find your own beliefs."

That was the encouragement I needed, and it's why I didn't just take his word for it when I called him about the toothache. Talking with him, as someone who had been in my shoes and made it to the other side, gave me so much hope.

When something as big as cancer shows up in your life, "impossible" comes up a lot. Everything feels impossible. The odds are just too great, and the territory is too unknown. If you think too much about it, you might feel the same way about starting a business or losing weight, or anything you might be struggling to overcome. Looking straight ahead at all that's left to do is overwhelming.

Talking to Greg helped me get the perspective of someone who's already past it and is looking back at all they've done. It's like someone who has climbed Mount Everest or won a championship. The only people who make it are the ones who focus on one step at a time. When they get done, they can look back and see how far they've come. The coach of the Washington Huskies women's basketball program was asked how they made it to the Final Four in 2016. He said, "We tried to win every shootaround, every bus ride, every walkthrough, every flight. We tried to win every single thing."

They had a 0.2 percent chance of making it that far. If making it had been their only goal, it wouldn't have happened. The odds are too great.

I read that quote while lying on my parents' couch, not long after the diagnosis, sitting with a 1 percent chance of outliving projections.

That team did whatever they could to win whatever they faced. Greg did whatever it took to take care of his body and live beyond his prognosis. I had to do the same.

Bad news, grim outcomes, and low odds are overwhelming. They make it seem impossible to reach our goals. They try to keep us focused on the huge task ahead rather than all of the little steps that can get us past it. But Nelson Mandela was exactly right: "It always seems impossible until it's done." If you can shift your mindset from the impossible odds to the steps you can take, you can break free of those limitations. You can focus on what's possible to do and then do it.

People who have made it to the other side know that to be true, and they become a light in the darkness. We need to hear more stories of people who have lived beyond cancer.

Who have built their small businesses. Who have changed their bodies, their mindset, and their lives. It's all too easy to talk about bad news and bad beats. Instead, talk about what you learned when you took a risk. Talk about how you've reframed that challenge. Talk about trying to win every moment, take one step at a time, change one habit that will get you closer. And when you're stuck in your room late at night, crying in a corner because the task ahead is so daunting, look for the light. Listen for the encouragers. We know what's possible. We want you to make it to the other side to know it too.

"Impossible" isn't real. It's a mindset, which means we can hang on to it or let it go. Dwelling on the impossible directs our energy toward resistance. It drags us down, and it usually drags the people around us down too. Like all mindsets, it's also contagious. We can spread our fear and negativity, like I found with some doctors and teachers and experts. Or we can let our vision outweigh the doubt and instead spread hope and encouragement.

We're all human. It's normal for humans to doubt and have fears. It's uncommon for us to face those fears and go after our dreams anyway. Choose the uncommon path, find people to join you on that path, and together take one step at a time until you've accomplished the impossible.

OBSTACLE

noun. a thing that blocks one's way or prevents or hinders progress.

synonyms: barrier, hurdle, problem, disadvantage.

I've said the word "obstacle" a lot, because it's something that we can expect to overcome. A barrier might block our way entirely, a setback can reverse progress, but an obstacle is something to move beyond. Unfortunately, when something seems difficult or impossible, we don't think of it as an obstacle. It becomes a problem, a struggle, or a barrier. It's easy to talk about these and to wallow in how difficult it is to face them. It's much harder to take action. And obstacles demand action.

In *Millionaire Success Habits*, Dean Graziosi talks about

turning success into daily habits rather than overall goals. The hard work comes every single day, with every single risk, every single obstacle. It's less like climbing over a wall and more like building a ladder, one piece at a time.

It's important to get clear on the words and perspective we use, because the way we talk about obstacles influences our approach and influences the people around us. Dean wrote about how the people in our lives tend to influence us toward playing it safe and staying where we are. It's usually well-meaning. They want to be nice. They don't want to see us fail. So they say things like "It's too difficult to get that position. Why not focus on what your degree is for?" or "That market is too competitive," or "Keep that job because it's secure," or "Go have a beer and a burger and enjoy your life."

You can really notice this in the difference between people who have taken action and people who haven't.

People who have taken action know what a gift failure can be. They know how much you can learn by trying to overcome that obstacle. The question is less about *can* you take the risk, and more about if you take the risk, what would you learn? I'm sure Steve Jobs had someone telling him to give it up or play it safe. If he had, Apple wouldn't be what it is today.

It's in the pursuit of goals, in the way we confront our obstacles, that we grow and develop as people. We learn who we are when we're pursuing our goals, failing, and trying again. All of the risk and lessons along the way add up to the vision you're pursuing. Making a million dollars isn't your obstacle—taking the first step toward it is. You'll either succeed or learn, and either way you win.

The uncommon path embraces failure. Thomas Edison famously said, "I have not failed. I've just found 10,000 ways that won't work." When your vision outweighs your fear of losing, that's when you become truly invincible. I thought invincibility was about nothing bad ever happening to me, when really it was about my ability to overcome whatever came my way. When you want something so badly that nothing can slow you down, it becomes true. Nothing can stop you; it can only teach you lessons.

FINISH STRONG

NOTHING IS IMPOSSIBLE

"Becoming is better than being."

—CAROL DWECK, *MINDSET: THE NEW PSYCHOLOGY OF SUCCESS*

* * *

Writing the Book

I am becoming my best self.

* * *

BELIEVE

verb. accept something as true; feel sure of the truth of.

Thinking back to the two surgeons who set me on my journey, it wasn't just their bedside manner or their perspective that made them so different from each other. It was their level of belief. The first surgeon decided from the very beginning that he wouldn't be successful. Even in my business, it's hard for me to work with someone who doesn't believe in themselves. How could I trust him when my life was on the line?

We all determine the path we're going to take. We decide on our destination, our limits, and whether or not we will keep moving forward. The surgeon who removed my tumor didn't place limitations on himself. He knew what he was capable of and believed in what was possible.

Ezra Pound once said, "What matters is not the idea a man holds, but the depth at which he holds it."

How are you holding your vision? How are you holding your challenge? It's important to set goals and have objectives, but if you're holding on to them loosely, shallowly, you'll let go of them as soon as things get difficult. You'll limit yourself, like the first surgeon who couldn't see beyond the ways things could go wrong.

Lying on that stretcher, being wheeled away from my family and into the halls toward the operating room, I felt like I was at my own funeral and they were pulling me to my grave. Because of the belief that my surgeon had and the confidence he gave to me, I was able to take a deep breath and trust that I would come back out later that night.

If you're surrounded by shallow belief, closed mindsets, scarcity, and doubt, that's what you'll absorb. If your belief isn't strong, that's what you'll convey to others. We can't do any of this alone. We're all connected to each other and affect each other. Pay attention to the voices that influence you and how you influence others.

We express doubt or belief every moment of every day. Not just when the big challenges come, but in each habit and routine that builds toward something bigger. To hang on to belief, you have to catch a vision so strong that you can see exactly where you're going and why. Go after that vision relentlessly, so that nothing and no one can slow you down. Have courage, even in the face of impossible odds. Your level of belief will carry you to your goals and will encourage everyone around you to do the same.

I'm not in the same position of doubt and fear that I was in back when I met those surgeons. I've been through so much that beating cancer feels like a normal part of my day. But my vision stretches so far beyond just surviving that I'm always up against something new. Even writing this book made me second-guess whether I was good enough, whether I had anything to say, whether I'd experienced enough in my life to make it worth writing everything down.

When I stepped away from the big vision of best-seller lists and sales and being an author, I remembered why I wanted to tell my story in the first place. When Dr. Meyers told me to write a book, I only really cared about reaching one person. If one person could be changed by my story, then the time and energy would be worth it. So I stopped trying to write a best seller and started trying to share my story.

I wrote down a page a day. I took time off. I came back and wrote more. I kept going until what seemed impossible was actually just...done. I took baby steps until I'd done the uncommon thing and had written a book. Just like I'd taken one step at a time to change my diet and my body, or one step at a time to beat cancer. No one else could tell me how to do these things. No one else could give me permission. It all had to come from my heart, my vision, and my beliefs.

Stop waiting for permission. Stop waiting for circumstances to be perfect. If there's something you want, go after it. Hold deep beliefs. Don't let anything pull them away from you. Let them carry you into the future you've dreamed of building.

> Stop searching for yourself. There's not a better you out there, with better habits and beliefs, just waiting to be found. You have to create yourself. If there's something you want, a success you're driving toward, an obstacle you're facing, you're the only person who can make it happen. Stop comparing yourself to others, to your past self, or to your future self. Be your own CEO and make it happen. I believe that you can. Now you have to believe it too.

30

ACCOMPLISH

verb. achieve or complete successfully.

synonyms: fulfill, realize, attain, execute, complete, finish, do

March 6, 2019. Exactly three years since I hopped in the car to go to the gym and my whole world fell apart. This time, it's a Wednesday morning, and I'm in downtown Austin getting some work done at a coffee shop. I'm single. I'm not trying to get shredded. And I've been through more than I could have imagined. But I'm also a survivor. I'm an entrepreneur. And I'm working on a business that routinely changes people for the better.

The morning was as mundane as one can be when your office is a coffee shop and you've beaten brain cancer. Then Joey showed up.

Joey and I have been friends since middle school, and it's been great to be in touch again. I remember when we were in sixth grade, shooting around at the gym and playing pickup games. After a couple hours, I would be ready to go home and relax. Joey would stay and work on his skills. Joey taught me a lot about what it means to work hard, and today was no different.

We did some catching up for a while, made small talk, and just hung out. Then he told me about his plans for the weekend.

"Nick and I are going to do a Goggins challenge. Want in?"

The three of us had all read David Goggins's book *Can't Hurt Me*, where he talked about all he's overcome and how he challenges himself daily to create the best version of himself. He completed the Navy SEAL Hell Week three different times, cross-trained in other branches, has set pull-up world records, and has competed in some of the most difficult marathons in the world. The Goggins Challenge was to run fifty miles at once, and they invited me along.

I'm not a runner, or at least I haven't been since I did a little track in middle school. Working out isn't the same as training, and my focus had been on my inner health, my business, and staying in shape. I hadn't prepared physically or mentally for something that intense. But I heard the words coming out of my mouth before I could think twice: "Yeah, I'll be there."

Over the next few days, I had plenty of second thoughts. I thought about how little I'd trained, how I could get hurt, and how Sunday was my day to relax. Then I thought about telling Joey it was time to relax back when we were twelve. He'd always driven me toward my true potential. Was that what was happening now?

The day before, I ran into Joey at the apartment complex. He told me that Nick had been fighting a sickness and might not participate. "If I have to do this alone, I will. It's fine," he said.

I couldn't let that happen. I got up that morning and fed my mind all of the encouragement and belief I could find. I wanted to go for thirty miles, and I had to believe that was possible or it wouldn't have been worth getting out of bed.

Seven o'clock came fast, and when I got to the park both Joey and Nick were there and ready to go. We started off around the ten-mile track, ready to take ourselves to new personal heights.

The first five miles were great. It was a mild spring day,

so there were some clouds but not rain, a little sun but not a ton of heat. We ran through the humidity and some sprinkles, through the doubts and the pain. With the first lap down, I felt better than I'd anticipated. Completing ten miles felt like an accomplishment already, and happened faster than I thought it would. We grabbed water from the home base we'd set up at the starting point. Joey told us, "One step at a time, boys!" and that's what we did.

I thought about the steps I'd taken over the last three years. How even the big things, like going keto, were never the finish line. They were just steps along the way toward the new me, the stronger me, the me filled with hope and belief. When I'd think about how much of the run was left in front of us, I'd also think about how insurmountable it has seemed to beat cancer. The only way to do it is to think about the present moment. What am I doing now that will get me one step closer?

"You can slow down or walk, but don't stop," he encouraged. I thought about the moments when I'd wanted to give up, and how action always brought me back to my vision. I kept going, adopting college football coach Nick Saban's strategy for his team: with each step, I chanted in my mind *the process, the process, the process, the process.*

Two laps in, my body started to rebel. We ran out of water at our home base, and none of the water fountains around the trail were working. My calf muscles stopped responding properly, and every step felt like my ankles were snapping. My heart pounded and I became dizzy. I slowed down to a walk, almost dragging my body forward. *The process, the process, the process.*

I thought about the process that it took to carry me from naïve nineteen-year-old to the healthier, more whole, successful adult I was becoming. I thought about the risks I had to take and the doubts I had to overcome. I thought about the people who followed my brand and the struggles that they'd faced. When the road gets hard, do we get to give up? Do we just sit back and say it's too hard, I'm not ready, I'll just relax?

The process, the process, the process.

Jogging, walking, or crawling, I had that thirty-mile marker as my destination, and I had to get there. The starting line is always exciting, but few people keep going when they feel like shutting down. We don't like pain or fear or struggle. Only those who are willing to take the uncommon path stick around to see the finish line.

I stopped relying on my body for fuel and started using my mindset. My throat was parched and I still had five miles to go. I had to sustain myself on belief and on gratitude. Life had thrown me so many curveballs, but here I was, pushing my body to the limits with good friends on a beautiful day. When my legs felt like they might snap, I thought of a regular at the coffee shop I hang out in. He labors just to walk to and from the counter, but he's never complaining or whining. That's his everyday life—how could I give up with just a little bit to go?

I made it back to our base and crossed the thirty-mile marker with my body in pain and my mind soaring. It was the most painful day of my life, as well as the most accomplished I've ever felt. I didn't do it for a plaque on the wall or bragging rights. I did it to take myself to new physical heights. I did it to challenge myself mentally and emotionally.

I did it because beating cancer wasn't enough. Reacting or surviving isn't enough. I have a vision. You have a vision. You have an incredible future. Focus on the process. Build a better version of yourself. It only seems impossible until it's done.

Most of us have run from our past. Some of us are running toward our future. But how many of us can just sit with the present? Every single moment that we have is beautiful and precious and worth investing in, even when it's painful.

We've all got a path to go down. We've all got a vision to realize. Build your belief up until the obstacles become beautiful, failure becomes a gift, and life becomes an incredible journey. You're the CEO of your own life. What are you going to do with it?

CONCLUSION

DEAR CANCER

I never thought I would meet you personally. As a kid, I thought I knew who you were. I would hear about friends and family members meeting you. I heard about how you destroyed lives—how you took lives.

I thought my life was too good for you.

When I met you, I realized just how fragile we are and how powerful you can be. You've hurt a lot of people, Cancer. You've taken lives, destroyed families, caused depression and anxiety, and stolen hope.

I forgive you, Cancer.

Not because you're gone. I'll never know if you're gone, actually. I might never know. But I forgive you.

You knew me long before I knew you. I wanted to pretend like you were new, like you hadn't been hiding and waiting, but you were there. I forgive myself for ignoring you.

I forgive you because I wouldn't be who I am today if we hadn't met. I know now that I didn't think that I was too good for you—I actually valued my life more than others. Without you teaching me that lesson, I wouldn't be able to help people the way I do now. I wouldn't have gained control over my own life, wouldn't have connected with other people, wouldn't have seen how strong we can all be.

While we're at it, thank you for introducing me to Time. We'd never been friends before. I never wanted to wait, never valued what Time had to offer. You helped me shake hands with Time...and with Fear, and Doubt...and my life is better for it.

Thank you for making me realize that life is a gift. Thank you for making me create happiness in my life. Thank you for making me grow.

I know people hate you, Cancer, and I can understand why. You're powerful, but you're not in control. Your darkness has made me realize that nothing is impossible. I'm going to keep telling the world you're not in control, and you're going to lose some power.

I hope you can forgive me for that, because it's my new mission, and it will happen.

Thank you, Cancer.

LOGAN

ACKNOWLEDGMENTS

Mom, you have done more for me than anyone in my life. I have been able to grow in so many ways because of what you have done for me—things I overlook. You gave me the faith that I have as soon as we left the hospital after the diagnosis. I wouldn't be here without you.

Dad, you have been my best friend my whole life. You have been there through thick and thin, every failure and success that I have experienced. Every day you give me the faith that is needed to achieve the impossible. Never have you let my faith fade away, and you always help me build my vision one step at a time.

Tyler, you have shown me what it means to create. Creating the best version of myself and the support you have shown me has helped me create change, create growth, and create a vision. Your art as a person is helping me carve the path in front of me.

Cayden, you will achieve so many amazing things in your life. Ever since you were born, you have brought so much joy to my life. You have a personality of never slowing down and being relentless. Your journey has only begun!

I want to personally thank every single person that has been there for me, has supported me, and has impacted my life. You know who you are, and I want to thank you all face to face. Every single supporter over social media, in person, and more, I can't thank you enough. Without each and every one of you, I would not be the person that I am today. I would not be where I am in my life. Because you all have impacted my life, I am able to impact thousands—millions! It isn't that I am changing lives, it's that we are all changing lives together. Thank you.

ABOUT THE AUTHOR

LOGAN SNEED is a brain cancer survivor and entrepreneur whose online business generated a six-figure income before his 21st birthday. A stage-4 cancer diagnosis didn't derail Logan's desire to reinvent himself every day and pursue the dreams he wasn't ready to give up. Today, Logan is an inspirational public speaker, social media influencer, ketogenic diet expert, and a best-self coach with a passion for personal transformation. To learn more or connect with Logan, visit LoganSneed.com.

.

Printed in Great Britain
by Amazon